THE COMPLEX LIFE OF A WOMAN DOCTOR

MEDICINE AND MOTHERHOOD

GLORIA O. SCHRAGER, M.D.

To order additional copies of this book, contact:
Xlibris Corporation
1-888-795-4274
www.Xlibris.com
Orders@Xlibris.com
32753

I believe it is difficult for those who publish their own memoirs to escape the imputation of vanity. Nor is this the only disadvantage under which they labour: it is also their misfortune, that whatever is uncommon is rarely, if ever, believed, and from what is obvious we are apt to turn with disgust, and to charge the writer of it with impertinence. People generally think those memoirs only worthy to be read or remembered which abound in great or striking events: those, in short, which in a high degree, excite either admiration or pity: all others they consign to contempt or oblivion.

(Olaudah Equiano, also known as Gustavus Vassa, written June 1792; republished in the *Classic Slave Narratives*, edited by Henry Louis Gates, Jr., 2002)

DEDICATION

For my grandchildren: Josh, Ben, Elana and Alec, and their parents: Luke and Frances, Ralph and Debbie, with much

ACKNOWLEDGEMENTS

M y thanks to Gene Brewer, an exacting editor and constant source of encouragement; to Rita Charon, MD, PhD, Professor and Director of Narrative Medicine at Columbia, whose charismatic leadership stimulated the writing of this book; to John Robison, my former patient and present computer wiz, who made endless housecalls during my computer emergencies; and of course to my wonderful family, who have always been there for me. My special thanks to my daughter-in-law, Frances Marshall, who urged me to write this memoir for my grandchildren.

CONTENTS

All the main characters in this book are accurately named. The names of patients, doctors and others who are identified by first names or initials have been changed to protect their privacy.

Introduction

I read Gloria Schrager's memoir of her many lives—student, pediatrician, wife and mother, health activist, powerful academic leader, grandmother, widow—with deep affection and tearful pride. I am fortunate to be Dr. Schrager's colleague at Columbia, our paths as women doctors crossing in committee work and educational efforts and cultural projects. Knowing her best through her participation in our medical center literature seminar as an astute and daring reader, I am not surprised at her fluency, her interpretive power, and her commanding skill as a story-teller. What I am not prepared for are her tremendous accomplishments. This modest pediatrician never revealed, much less boasted of, all that she has done. The first Director of Pediatrics at Overlook Hospital, an influential affiliated teaching hospital of Columbia University, at that time, Dr. Schrager wielded her powerful and irrevocable will to launch a teaching pediatric service, a pediatric residency program, a pediatric sub-specialty service, a neonatal intensive care unit, and countless major advances in the care of ill infants and children. She created a stellar academic department of pediatrics quite literally from the ground up, engaging her colleagues, trustees, donors, hospital executives, parents and patients with her generosity and her vision.

Dr. Schrager undertook the writing of this memoir as a service to women physicians, including her niece and grandniece. She wanted us to know what led up to our relative ease in entering the medical profession. We women doctors who entered medical schools after the mid-1970s walked a way paved by our foremothers. We were not barred from residencies, as was Dr. Schrager. We were not assumed to be nurses or patients on walking onto hospital wards, as was Dr. Schrager. We had freedoms won in costly battles by these brave and lonely women who came before us. How enraging to read of the blatant sexism confronted by our protagonist. How moving to witness her steady determination to win respect and equity—not only for herself but for those she knew would follow her. That her students and residents adore and respect her is no surprise—she enacts medicine's ideals of clinical astuteness, professionalism, and humanism without show, without calling attention to herself. In the course of this account, readers learn of her lucky and brilliant diagnostic coups and her ability to stick to her guns when she knows the right thing to do. We learn also of her deeply regretted clinical mistakes or miscalculations, this author with the humility to look squarely at all aspects of her life in medicine. Dr. Schrager's commitment to her calling is staggering, and her shrewdness and diplomacy in achieving her goals breath-taking.

The Complex Life of a Woman Doctor tells the story of a Jewish girl, born to second-generation immigrant parents in1924 in Brooklyn and raised in down-at-the-heels rural up-state New York, who endures poverty and solitude to create a life of independence and influence. Her mother works as an embroiderer in the factory that was the site of the deadly Triangle Fire of 1911, escaping death by having stopped working only a few months before the conflagration. Her father's prosperity as one of the first Chrysler dealers crashes in the Great Depression of 1929. Despite financial hardships, her parents' and older brothers' unconditional love give her tremendous confidence and freedom and sense of worth. The Dickensian bleakness of her aunt's grudging and demeaning care, necessary during especially rough times in the family, marks the young Gloria with a fierceness for self-sufficiency. Anti-Semitism of the early Nazi years reaches into the Adirondacks town. The Spanish Civil War erupts. Pearl Harbor is bombed. Paul Robeson sings in a Black church in Philadelphia, Gloria the only white person in the audience. McCarthy witch-hunts cost her brother his position as university professor. The women's movement, the Vietnam war, the Newark riots, the 1960s drug scene, Benjamin Spock's presidential bid—all these major life-changing events unfold within our narrative as both backdrop and powerful influences on the life of our protagonist.

This work achieves the aims of memoir—brilliantly—by registering and interpreting the major world events that participate in and are inflected by the local events of this individual life. The life story of a girl destined to become a powerful physician tells the story of a nation divided by racism and misogyny. It tells the story of a world haunted by Hitler's anti-Semitism and of the war that was necessary to stop him. It tells the story of a medicine that gradually, if reluctantly, embraces its women practitioners, that develops the knowledge and power to care for sick children stricken with polio, tuberculosis, congenital heart disease, leukemia, renal failure, strokes. The author knows that her trajectory tells more than her own story, that its compass exceeds individual choices and preferences. She was called—it was simply her time and place—to participate in events of national and professional and international gravity. What she did—and this was given to her—*mattered* in widening circles of consequence for the country and the profession and the world.

And so, she responded with conscience and summoned up the duty to answer that call, not only to live the life but to tell it. I know that our author had to surmount the scruples of modesty; she had to quiet the uneasy belief that publication was unseemly, for it is not in her nature to place herself on display. Her sense of duty overcame her private doubts, and for that we are most grateful. She chooses as epigraph a citation from Olaudah Equiano's 1792 slave narrative: "People generally think those memoirs only worthy to be read or remembered which abound in great or striking events: those, in short, which in a high degree, excite either admiration or pity: all others they consign to contempt or oblivion." What an honest *mise-en-scène* for one's memoir—to admit that one does not know with certainty what is striking, what admirable, what worthy of contempt. The sign of this work's authenticity and power is that the great and striking events described here make seamless weave with the private ones. The great and striking events do not emerge automatically or inevitably but rather unfold as the consequence of many individuals' choices and courage. The public is but the private collated, and this private individual has the clarity of sight to recognize and fulfill her responsibilities as an agent and recorder of change.

Dr. Schrager writes with warmth and directness. She tells her story plainly and with authority. Her control is enviable. Even in stretches detailing horribly insulting treatment by misogynist or anti-Semitic supervisors or colleagues, the author maintains the grace and tact to prevail. She prevails—by virtue not only of her nerve and wit but also by virtue of her deep commitment to the needs of patients and her love of medicine. Written for a lay audience, this book teaches its readers across a very wide range of subjects—human genetics, bacteriology, human physiology, child-rearing practices—while instructing in the power of patience, dignity, and confidence in one's mission.

The memoir is a love story of passion and depth. Gloria's long marriage to Al Schrager is the frame for all her accomplishments. They meet as interns at Metropolitan Hospital, fall in tempestuous love, survive a stormy courtship, and mature into a nuanced, witty, generative marriage that seems the magnetic center for the billowing extended family that evolves. Pictures accompanying the text show handsome young men, pretty young women, cousins and in-laws and grandchildren, seemingly protected and nourished within the orbit of a muscular, certain love. Husband's and wife's professional lives are entwined: working out of one office in their home while raising their two boys, internist Dr. Al and pediatrician Dr. Gloria do house calls, care for neighbors and friends, attend at all hours to patients who show up at the office for care. The core story here that lends meaning to the professional and scientific and political and moral stories is the account of this remarkable family. With such zest to do they go on family trips and rent Tuscan villas and walk the Great Wall and return over and over to their beloved Paris. With resolve and familial strength, they see one child through Hodgkin's Disease and its treatment. They take in aging parents, various ill or down-on-their-luck relatives, never saying no, always making room, ever loyal and, yes, in love all their lives.

Al dies of a sudden heart attack. Gloria is inconsolable, but responds with her characteristically vehement grasp on her independence. She soldiers on in the home they made together, not giving in to children's pleas to move in with them. The author deftly describes this most difficult passage in her life, not sentimentalizing her loss but placing it squarely in front of the reader to behold in its complexity. She brings readers through her breast cancer and treatment, her long grieving, her continued zeal for advances in pediatric care, preventive public health, and equitable health care.

Accompanying the author's text are two accounts by the women doctors in her family—her older brother's daughter Barbara and her grandniece Rebecca. This is the heritage. This is the immediate lineage, and it is through the words and reflections of the next two generations of women doctors that we take the measure of the greatness of this work and this life. Courage comes to us from many sources, and one source can provide many with courage. As Dr. Schrager's colleague at Columbia, I derive tremendous nourishment from simply knowing her, witnessing her poise and wit, learning from her close readings of Kafka's "Metamorphosis" or Joyce's "The Dead," taking in all that she and her cohort of women doctors did for me and for our beloved medicine. I revel in this remarkable incarnation of the steely goodness possible in medicine, the unswerving insistence on justice and effectiveness. This is what medicine—and life—are about, I can see with the illumination of Gloria Schrager's life, this authenticity, this wide and deep knowledge of health and suffering, this unconditional love, this joy in a life that counts.

Rita Charon, MD, PhD
Professor of Clinical Medicine
Director, Program in Narrative Medicine
College of Physicians and Surgeons
of Columbia University

CHAPTER ONE

The Beginnings

I decided to become a doctor on a Friday, at precisely 3:30 PM. The year was 1942 and I was a college sophomore majoring in history while living through one of history's most cataclysmic events. We were in the midst of World War II and I found my courses, particularly our heated dialectic discussions about the Industrial Revolution, of capitalism versus Marxism, increasingly irrelevant.

Most of my fellow students were divided into different factions, each with strong beliefs about the future of society. The Trotskyites and Stalinists hated capitalism, but they hated each other more. Socialists hated them both, but had only vague utopian ideas to offer as an alternative. And of course they all turned on the few who dared defend capitalism. All these groups would argue violently, their raised voices and gesticulations continuing after the end of class, spilling out into the corridors and down to the cafeteria, repeated day after day. I lost interest. They seemed to miss a vital point: there would be no future for any of this idealism if Hitler won the war. And in those dark days, this seemed a distinct possibility.

Science offered a more attractive source for learning and the next semester I elected to take some science courses, principally biology and chemistry. My biology professor, Dr. Alexander Novikoff, taught by the Socratic method. This was a new experience for me. Of medium height, he still seemed to tower over his terrified class as he paced back and forth like a caged tiger, hands clasped behind the back of his stained lab coat, suddenly stopping to pounce on some luckless student. His penetrating questions and his ironic way of dragging the answers from us forced us to think and reason independently, rather than be passive recipients of his knowledge. His owl-like horn rimmed glasses didn't hide the amusement in those piercing black eyes. He was obviously enjoying himself, sometimes stroking his bristling black moustache when gratified by a student's response.

Some of the students said resentfully that he was a sadist. To my surprise, I found I was beginning to enjoy the class and would occasionally even see the humor in his method. Although usually a silent participant in my courses, I began to challenge him and often found that Novikoff and I had entered in a dialogue. The rest of the class didn't seem to mind: they were relieved to have a brief respite from his eternal questioning.

One day, Novikoff asked me to help him with some research. He had just acquired an electron microscope—still considered a new and revolutionary invention—and was investigating the various structures in the cell, revealed in such startling detail by this powerful new technology. My job was making cell preparations from various plants, to be examined under the microscope. We would then photograph the images and speculate about the significance of the discoveries revealed in this new ultramicroscopic world we had entered. After several months, on that fateful Friday afternoon, he suggested that I switch my major to the sciences and continue with research.

I wasn't ready for this. In great awe of the man, I was both astonished and flattered by his suggestion, and yet, and yet— the thought of spending my life in a laboratory just didn't appeal to me. For a few moments I sat quietly, thinking of what to say, reluctant to hurt or anger him in any way.

He looked at me with his keen, perceptive eyes. "Not so enthusiastic about a career spent staring into a microscope?" His laugh was understanding but rueful.

"I'm not sure" I said. "A lab can be a lonely place. I think I'd like to work with people."

He nodded. "I get your point. You'd probably go nuts cooped up in a place like this for long periods of time."

"You didn't go nuts."

"Who says?" He chuckled, with a sparkle in his eyes that created a special sense of pleasure in the quiet lab.

"All right then," I said as he removed his glasses and wiped his eyes, still smiling. "Let's say you're right. What do you think I should do?"

He sighed and sat back on his tall stool, leaning his elbows on the lab bench behind him. "I'm afraid that's your call," he said, his face and voice suddenly serious. "What are you thinking about?"

What was I thinking about? I really had no idea. But I was grimly determined to find some line of work that would make me totally independent, not only financially but also free of superiors to contend with. I had had my fill of any number of part-time jobs as waitress, sales girl and file clerk and had gotten the unpleasant taste of office politics that I wanted to avoid in the future. I shrugged my shoulders.

Novikoff looked at me speculatively. "You know, with your aptitude for science and your interest in people, perhaps you should consider becoming a doctor."

"But women don't become doctors, they become nurses."

"Nonsense. Of course there are women doctors. I think you'd be a very good one. Why don't you apply to medical school?"

It would be nice to say that at that moment I had an epiphany: that I heard heavenly voices calling me to succor suffering humanity. Certainly the prospect of helping people was appealing, but the driving force behind my instant decision was more personal. It represented a way to achieve goals that had eluded me so far: independence and respect. To understand how important these goals were to me, how grimly determined I was to achieve them over all obstacles, I have to recount something of my bizarre childhood.

It started off conventionally enough. I was the youngest child born to Russian Jewish immigrants. My father, Ellis M. Ogur, and my mother, Edith Levine, had come to the United States as teenagers; my father at eighteen, my mother at sixteen, in 1906 and 1908 respectively. Their families were related and they had met at a large family function. In those days, many marriages were arranged, and even though they were not forced into this match, both families strongly encouraged it. Their wedding in 1911 was celebrated in typical Jewish style by a huge host of relatives from the combined families.

Neither had the time or opportunity to obtain any formal education in this country, since they had to earn a living. They could read and write fluently in Yiddish and Russian, each of which had a different alphabet. English meant learning a third alphabet as well as a third language but they taught themselves to do it. Their writing had the careful, stilted look of fine script. Their letters, even to members of the family, were always very formal.

My mother did embroidery and made lace in the building that was the scene of the notorious Triangle Fire in 1911. She had stopped working there, to get married, just a few months before the disaster. My father worked in construction, which was his father's trade in Russia. They made every effort to become thoroughly Americanized and spoke only English to their children. When they wanted to keep something secret from us, they spoke in Yiddish. It didn't work very well. All of us learned to understand Yiddish just by exposure to the language.

I had two brothers considerably older than I. My parents had wanted a little girl, "eine maidele," for some time and were overjoyed when my mother became pregnant again after a lapse of many years.

There were many family stories, repeated many times, about my birth. It occurred on a Friday. My mother was preparing for the Sabbath and as she felt the onset of labor, she rushed to finish cleaning the house and baking cakes "for the company" that would be visiting to see the new baby. I was born at home in a brownstone that my parents owned on Eastern Parkway, a beautiful tree-lined boulevard, in Brooklyn. I was the last of their three children. The family doctor who delivered me was a good friend of my parents and his first words to my mother were "Mazel tov! Du hast eine maidele—mit dimples!" Those dimples—cute in a little girl—became something of a handicap later in life. Sometimes, people found it difficult to take seriously a grown woman with dimples.

My parents considered the date of my birth, 7/11/24, quite propitious. Most of the men in our family did a modest amount of gambling, and the combination 7/11 was thought to be particularly lucky. And indeed things seemed to go well. I was a chubby rambunctious little girl with big dark eyes and a thick curly mop of hair. My adoring parents wanted to have a professional picture taken when I was about two, but I kept bouncing around on the special little armchair made for children's portraits. The exhausted photographer finally got my picture sitting backwards on the chair, legs astride. They kept it, in an elaborate golden frame, above their bed for years.

My father had taught himself to drive and was the first person in our extended family to buy a car, an elegant Pierce Arrow that was his particular pride. He had it for many years. I remember it well. It had monstrous trumpet-like headlights and a claxon horn that was deafening. The car stood quite high and had a running board, making it easier to step up into the seats. As children, we loved to stand on it, hanging on to the door and whooping and cheering while my father slowly drove the car a short distance to give us a special thrill. The rear windows had shades with little fringes on them, and attached to the sides of the rear doors were small vases for flowers. The engine had to be started with a crank that was inserted into the front of car and took a considerable amount of strength to turn. It usually took repeated attempts before the engine "caught" and we held our breath while it sputtered and finally burst into a powerful roar, to cheers from the entire family.

All our relatives were quite impressed by this new acquisition, and my father polished it carefully each weekend. I still associate the smell of polish and leather with our long weekend drives. My father used to crowd as many people as possible into the car, the children sitting on the adults' laps, and take us all for a picnic. There were two folding jump seats, as well as the regular seat in back, so that as many as ten passengers, including the children, could squeeze in. I always tried to choose the lap of the person nearest the window so I could see out, keeping the window wide open to feel the fresh breeze on my face.

Our favorite picnic spot was a park on Long Island near a gently flowing brook, in the shade of a grove of weeping willows. In front of the trees was a field sprinkled with wild flowers where we children could run and play. One of my uncles had a ukulele and another a balalaika, and everyone sang the popular songs of the day ("A Bicycle Built for Two" and "He Married the Girl with the Strawberry Curl") as well as many Russian folk songs. Some of the folk songs were melancholy, but the picnics were merry affairs. I remember picking wild flowers to put into the little vases that hung by the back seat of the car.

My father had met Mr. Chrysler, who had just started his own company manufacturing cars, and Dad became one of the first automobile dealers for Chrysler in the New York metropolitan area. Business was thriving and he invested heavily in expansion. And then came 1929 and the start of the Depression. The business failed and he was advised to declare bankruptcy. Stubborn and proud, he refused to do this and paid off all his creditors, selling our home and leaving us destitute. He had a large amount of Chrysler stock that he considered valueless. He gave the certificates to us for play money. I wonder what that stock would be worth today if we had saved it.

The run of bad luck continued in 1930 when I was bitten by a bulldog while skating down a city street. He clamped his jaws in my leg and had to be forcibly removed. After the initial fright, I seemed fine until several days later. When I tried to get up from dinner one evening, I found I couldn't stand on the affected leg. My parents, thinking I had sat on it curled under me, tried to massage it and the leg went into excruciatingly painful spasms. These became more frequent and more severe over the next weeks. The slightest vibration in the house would cause my leg to react. I became critically ill and my parents called in specialists they could ill afford. None of them could diagnose the problem. They considered rabies, or an allergic reaction to the tetanus shot I had received, or hysteria. The one thing they all agreed on was that my chances for survival were slim. (Years later, I discovered the diagnosis serendipitously in medical school. It was probably a form of local tetanus. The shot I had received was enough to prevent the spread of the toxin throughout my body but was inadequate to counteract the higher concentrations of toxin around the dog bite.)

When I began to recover weeks later, I was very weak. My parents were still worried about me and my father wanted to get out of the city to a place where there would be sunshine and fresh air to restore my health and where he could make a fresh start. He had begun to hate the city with its long bread lines and soup kitchens. There was no work to be had. Depression described not only the economy, but the faces of the crowds of unemployed.

To the surprise and consternation of the family, he loaded the Pierce Arrow with supplies to last for a week's exploration and drove straight north until he was in the Adirondack Mountains, not far from the Canadian border. After a considerable search, he found a parcel of land for sale bordering a beautiful body of water, Schroon Lake. There was a deserted gas station on the property. The land, about four acres, was very marshy. The lake flooded up to the road in springtime when the ice melted, inundating a good portion of it. It was generally considered uninhabitable.

The owners were anxious to get rid of it and told my father he could buy it for little more than a thousand dollars. But he didn't have the money or collateral for a mortgage. He asked his sister, the wife of a prosperous pharmacist, for a loan but she (and the rest of the family) thought he had taken leave of his senses. When she realized he was determined to leave the city, she finally agreed with great reluctance to advance the minimal amount required for a down payment. And so, with all our belongings packed into the back of the Pierce Arrow, we moved in early spring of 1931 to our new home. My brothers, both of whom were attending Brooklyn College, would join us for summer vacations and holidays. They were sent to live with my aunt until the end of the school year. Maurice (Moe) was ten years older than I. Tall and athletic, he greatly resembled my father with his dark good looks. He was a serious, taciturn young man and a brilliant student. Milton (Mickey), eight years my senior, was more like my mother. He was shorter and fair-skinned with light hazel eyes and brown curly hair. He had a sunny, pleasant disposition, a marvelous sense of humor and a love of music. He was something of a dreamer, not as involved with his studies, causing my parents some anxiety.

This was the first time I had been separated from my brothers whom I adored. I began to miss them as soon as we waved our goodbyes. I pressed my nose against the car window, waving until we were out of sight, and burst into tears. My mother silently dabbed her eyes with a handkerchief. My father stared grimly ahead. It was a dismal start to our journey. The trip took over twelve hours along the rutted, potholed Route 9, in bad condition because of the winter freeze. The superhighways of today did not exist. We had two flat tires that delayed us even more because my father had to partially unload the heavily laden car so he could jack it up to change the tires. We couldn't make the trip in one day and stopped for the night in Saratoga Springs. It was like a ghost town during the Depression. Most of the grand old hotels were boarded up. We stayed at a shabby boarding house run by an elderly couple. They looked at us with open scorn as we climbed wearily out of the car, travel-worn and rumpled. The man eyed the car, packed to the roof with our household belongings. "Never thought I'd see Okies in this part of the country," he drawled. He made my father pay in advance before he would even show us a room. ("Okies" referred to the Oklahoma share-croppers who were leaving their drought-stricken state in their battered jalopies and migrating to California with all their worldly goods. John Steinbeck describes them poignantly in *The Grapes of Wrath*.) We left Saratoga before dawn.

Snowdrifts were still piled along the side of the shack that was to be our new home. It had no insulation or indoor plumbing. The wind whistled through it. The nights were particularly cold and dreadful. We could hear bears knocking over the garbage cans outside, just a few feet away. I was not quite seven years old and I was terrified that they would come crashing through the flimsy walls and attack us. I was even more miserable because I knew that my mother was unhappy with the decision to move out of the city. As poor as we had become, she still had the comfort of a warm circle of family and friends, and she missed them. Living in a shack in virtual wilderness, where even the nearest neighbors were a distance away and not of her religion or background, was a severe culture shock

My father's first task was to construct a solid main building. As a young man in Russia he had helped his father, a builder and tinsmith, and he had not forgotten the skills. By the opening of the summer tourist season our new home was just about finished. It consisted of a long, narrow dining room where my mother ran a restaurant single-handed. The kitchen and bathroom were in the back. We slept in the unfinished attic above the kitchen. My father made a deal with the Gulf Oil Company to refurbish the gas station, providing us with additional income.

My mother had only cooked for her own family, but now she had to do it as a business. We visited other restaurants, where she would stealthily copy the menus and prices while we ordered something cheap—usually a grilled cheese sandwich, which cost ten cents. She wrote her own menus by hand, puzzling over what to charge. My father said a steak dinner should cost a dollar but she felt that was too much. They compromised on ninety-five cents. The dinner included soup, two vegetables, dessert and coffee. It was a while before they began to keep an account of the many costs of running a restaurant and adjust their prices accordingly. Although my father had some business experience with his car dealership, running a restaurant was quite different. It was my brother Moe who made my parents realize that, in addition to the money they spent to buy food, they had to consider the many hidden costs of equipment, maintenance, wood for the fire, etc.

The change that took place in my mother's personality was astonishing. In Brooklyn, she had been the obedient housewife, totally dependent on her husband the breadwinner. Now she was an equal partner in a business venture that was hazardous but necessary. She had always been shy, aware of her foreign accent and reluctant to speak with people outside the family circle, especially "Yankees." Now she was surrounded by them and had to learn their strange customs and dietary habits. I remember the first time someone came into the restaurant and asked for a western egg sandwich. She replied apologetically, "I'm sorry, we only have eastern eggs."

Fortunately, the man thought she was joking and laughed heartily. She smiled and her innate sense of humor began to assert itself. She was an attractive woman, slim, with green eyes that seemed to slant upwards when she smiled. Her long, wavy red hair reached almost to her waist when she brushed it out at night. During the day, she wore it in two thick coils covering her ears, like Princess Leia in *Star Wars*. She had a sense of style. She could twist a scarf or place a decorative pin to make the simple shirtwaists and skirts she wore to work look special.

The number of regular customers began to grow and included the state troopers who patrolled Route 9. They would roar up on their motorcycles for their midday meal and always ate two pieces of my mother's homemade pie. The restaurant became quite busy. My mother was an excellent cook, and she added side dishes from her Jewish cuisine that were unfamiliar up north—potato pancakes, chicken soup with matzoh balls (she called them dumplings), and sour cream. The latter engendered much speculation. She had to explain, when she served it on strawberries, that it wasn't whipped cream and had a different taste. But most took to it and tourists from the city flocked to the only restaurant in the area serving that kind of food. Undoubtedly it was her good cooking that attracted them all but as she became less shy she began to laugh and joke as she did with her family. That and the tantalizing aroma of freshly baked cakes and pies created a warm, friendly atmosphere.

Before long she needed help and Gerty Venner, a Schroon Lake native, came to work for us. Gerty was a large, capable, no-nonsense woman with faded blue eyes and graying brown hair that was always escaping in wisps from the severe bun she wore at the back of her head. She wore an enormous, flowered apron, immaculate because she changed it frequently. She kept a supply of them in the kitchen and in her spare time helped my mother with the laundry for the entire establishment, including the tourist cottages my father had begun to build and rent out.

Gerty was also an excellent cook and introduced my mother to new dishes. The most outstanding were Gerty's apple pies, not usually part of Jewish cuisine. They had a flaky, delicate crust that my mother soon learned to make. These homemade pies were one of the special attractions of the restaurant. Gerty brought a new dimension to the menu we served. In Brooklyn, we had kept a kosher home, as did the rest of my mother's family. My father's family was not observant. My mother had recognized that she could not keep kosher in Schroon Lake but had been reluctant to add ham or bacon to the menu. Gerty made her overcome such scruples. It was a difficult step for my mother to take but she saw the necessity of expanding her menu if she were to run a successful business. She never ate pork products herself. My brothers and I, running wild and barefoot, developed ravenous appetites and ate heartily of everything in the kitchen. It was always a cause for rejoicing when the college year ended and they were able to leave the city, and my aunt's house, to rejoin us at Schroon Lake.

Gerty worked for us for many years and became a close friend. She had a heavy, deliberate step and refused to be rushed, even when the restaurant was full and people were clamoring for service. She was very protective of my mother, who would become anxious and excited when the restaurant got busy. Gerty would say grumpily, "Don't let them upset you, ma'am. They know that good food takes time to prepare. If they're in a hurry, let them eat that swill up the road."

As my mother's self-confidence grew, she began to take a more active part in all business decisions. My father was a very stubborn man used to having his own way, and he was appalled by this change in his wife. While my mother had delicate features and a soft, musical voice, the temper usually associated with red hair suddenly became manifest. I wasn't used to their arguing. My mother had always had a sunny, pleasant disposition, loved to sing, and had deferred to my father on all family matters This new assertiveness angered him and their arguments grew heated.

"Please don't fight," I sobbed.

The three of us formed a tight little island in this strange, new, sometimes hostile environment and to a seven-year-old the threat that this too might come apart was frightening.

My mother, quite remorseful, took me in her arms and crooned, "Hush, dear. We weren't fighting."

The steely cold look in my father's eyes gradually disappeared and he muttered: "We were just discussing things. Everything's okay."

Dad, although not happy with this new aspect of his wife's character, was basically a very kind person and obviously loved my mother very much. I don't believe they ever went to bed mad at each other.

Bedtime was a challenge. We usually wore more flannel shirts and sweaters to bed than we wore during the day. The only heat in the house was from the large wood-burning stove my father bought for the kitchen. Its primary function was for the cooking and baking but we kept it going all night for warmth. Dad would buy a cord of wood and pile it near the back door. He or my brothers would split the wood with an axe so it could fit in the stove. My mother still spoke a lot of Yiddish and the cry "Hock Holtz"—chop wood—would echo through the house frequently. I was very fond of that stove and loved the smell of the burning wood, particularly when my father got a load of cedar for the fire. The fragrance would permeate the whole house, bringing a sense of comfort, particularly on cold nights. I would open the oven door and stick my feet in to get warm while I sat and read on a chair in front of the stove. Much later in life I saw similar stoves for sale in antique shops for astronomical prices, the same slogan proudly emblazoned on their cast-iron exteriors: "From Kalamazoo Direct to You."

The unfinished attic where we slept above the kitchen remained reasonably comfortable because of the heat rising from the stove. Toward morning, however, the fire would die out and it was freezing—literally. My father had a set of false teeth that he kept in a glass of water near his bed at night. I remember several occasions when he had to thaw the ice in the glass to get at his teeth.

In the morning, I would help my mother make up the shopping list for the day. We bought most of the produce for the restaurant from local farmers. I loved to go with my father to the farm owned by Mr. H. A tall, good-natured, grizzled man in overalls, he would come trudging out of the fields with a friendly wave and a big "Halloooo." My job was to collect the eggs from under the chickens. Then I would wander around while he and my father chatted and leisurely gathered the rest of the produce on our list. He had many dogs on his property and one day a half-grown puppy with silky brown and white fur and gentle brown eyes came bounding over to be petted, wagging his tail wildly. It was love at first sight. I pleaded to keep him and Mr. H., smiling at us, drawled, "I reckon your little girl needs that dawg more than I do." Mr. H. had already named him Carlo and was training him to retrieve the pheasants and grouse that farmers shot and smoked in their smokehouses for the winter.

Carlo was some kind of indeterminate breed, part collie, part retriever and incredibly smart. He seemed to understand everything. My father would spend the long cold nights teaching him intricate retrieving tricks. He would have Carlo smell some piece of clothing such as a glove or sock, then hide it somewhere in the room and tell Carlo to find it and return it to its owner. Carlo never failed.

Shortly after he joined our family, Carlo brought us a litter of newborn rabbits, their eyes still sealed shut. He carried them gently in his mouth one by one and deposited them at our feet. We couldn't find the nest or the mother and assumed she had been killed. My father made a cage for them. I fed them sugar water with an eyedropper and then diluted milk as they grew. When they graduated to shredded vegetables I released them in the back yard. They hopped away into the trees near the lake but would continue to come back often to be fed. Carlo never chased them, as he did the wild squirrels and raccoons who rummaged in the garbage. We kept him inside at night, when the bears came. Years later, when I was taking care of premature infants during my residency, I thought frequently of those baby rabbits.

When Dad was not teaching Carlo tricks during those long cold nights, he would be making beautiful objects out of hammered copper: plates, lamps and other ornaments. Dad was a skilled craftsman with a love for beauty. I still have some platters and a copper lamp that he made for me. He liked working with his hands. He was not much of a reader.

My mother loved to read. She was very concerned about world affairs and read the daily newspapers avidly. She also had a well-thumbed collection of Russian novels. They were by Turgenev, Tolstoy, Chekov and probably others. She would read them in the original Russian, occasionally forming the words soundlessly with her lips.

CHAPTER TWO

My Childhood at Schroon Lake

W hen we first moved to Schroon Lake in 1931, my schooling was considered of secondary importance. I was seven years old and had no formal education. That fall, my parents enrolled me in a little country school house about half a mile down the road. All elementary school grades were taught in one room on the first floor. Middle school and high school were upstairs. To this day, I don't understand how our elementary school teacher was able to teach all grades, keep discipline, and give each child special attention. She was a young French-Canadian woman with large, smiling dark eyes and expressive hands that seemed to dance as she taught. We mispronounced her name badly but she was very patient and didn't mind. She had an encouraging word for every child and I loved her.

The school was a picturesque white wooden frame building near the town cemetery, on top of a hill, with steps leading up from the road. The building was capped with a bell tower. The bell had a deep, resonant sound that echoed off the mountains and could be heard for miles. It used to ring twice before each school day—once for a ten-minute warning, and a second time as a late bell. We were about a 15 minute walk south of the school on old Route 9, and if I heard that warning bell, I would break all speed records to get there on time. That building is gone now. During the second Roosevelt administration, the WPA built a large, modern central school on the north side of town. It was over a mile from where we lived and I had to take the school bus. The hill where the little schoolhouse stood has been excavated. When I visited Schroon Lake years later, an ugly gas station with battered old pickup trucks, wrecked cars and piles of used tires was on that property. The back of the station abutted the raw earth of the excavation. I felt as if that lovely place

CHILDHOOD IN SCHROON LAKE

Mt. Pharaoh From Our Property

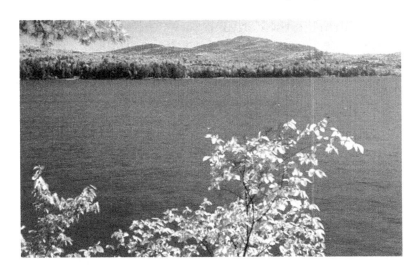

First Day of School 1932

Target Practice 1938

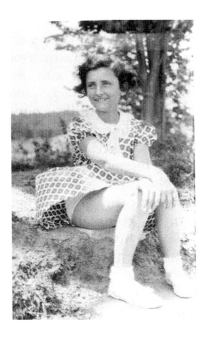

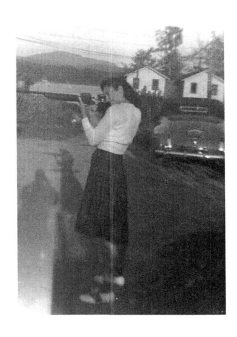

had been defiled. Much more had changed. The hill across the road from us, with its wild berry bushes, has become the site of a high-speed parkway, the Northway. It bisects the trails I hiked to the forests beyond. I wonder if the deer who used to come to the lake to drink in the early morning, their antlers reflected in the mirror-like waters, can still find their way there.

When I was attending the little schoolhouse, the children were bussed directly from school to their houses of worship for a half-day of religious instruction each week. I was the only Jew in the school and the nearest Jewish community was over 40 miles away, in Glens Falls. The school authorities didn't know what to do with me and decided that I should sit in the library during the afternoon reserved for religion. I became an avid reader and looked forward to that private time even though it emphasized my difference from the rest of the school.

Every Memorial Day the school held a pageant, followed by a parade down Main Street to the park, where the town band would play patriotic music (mostly marches by John Philip Sousa) and everyone would picnic on the lawn. When I was in the sixth grade my elementary school teacher picked me to play Lady Liberty and a boy in my class to be George Washington in the pageant that began the festivities. We had the major speaking roles. At the end, when the curtain came down, we all were supposed to scramble to form a tableau, with George Washington and Lady Liberty standing on stools like statues, he with one hand on his sword and the other tucked into his jacket like Napoleon; me with the torch of liberty raised high, while around us all the children in the school waved American flags and everyone joined us in singing "The Star Spangled Banner." George Washington was a hateful little boy named Heinrich with pale blue eyes and a blond crew cut. His father owned one of the stores in town and was openly sympathetic with Hitler. When his parents heard about the pageant, they complained about their son sharing the spotlight with a Jew, "who wasn't really an American." The school ignored them but when it came time for the Grand Finale of the pageant and we rushed to form the tableau, one of the stools we were to stand on had mysteriously disappeared. Both George Washington and I ran to the one remaining stool but he got there first and jumped up, looking down at me with a victorious smile, hand on sword, assuming his Napoleonic pose. I stood there for a moment uncertain what to do, then ran off stage, grabbed an American flag, and as the curtain went up, marched grandly back to stand in front of him, waving the torch of liberty and the flag high above me, effectively blocking him from view. My teacher was incensed, wanting to know who had removed the stool. The principal said with a grin, "Never mind. That little girl more than held her own."

These were the 1930's, during Hitler's rise to power. Anti-Semitism was flagrant and universal. Walking down the road to school I would pass boarding houses with signs on their neat front lawns: "No dogs or Jews allowed." Hitler's rantings were broadcast frequently on the radio. Radio reception was poor because we were in a valley between tall mountains but despite the static and difficulty in hearing, my parents listened intently, shaking their heads with worry. We still had many relatives in Europe. Closer to home, many noted Americans openly shared Hitler's hatred of the Jews. We had to listen to the frequent hate-filled sermons of Father Coughlin and the saccharine venom of Kate Smith, an obese, simpering woman who was a popular singer. Even our national hero, Charles Lindbergh, admired Hitler.

I had few friends except for a little girl who lived "down the road a piece." We became inseparable until the priest warned her family about the dire consequences of consorting with Jews. We then had to meet secretly and Ellie was in constant fear that the priest would find out. Several months later she developed pneumonia, was rushed to the hospital in Ticonderoga, and died. I was inconsolable and felt responsible. Her father, a sturdy French-Canadian who had become a friend of my father's despite the priest's warning, made a special trip to our house to talk to me. He asked me, as Ellie's best friend, to come to the wake. I was horrified at the idea of viewing my friend in a coffin but my father said it was important to show respect and he would take me. When I saw the wax-like figure, I thought, "That isn't Ellie, it's just a wax doll. She's played a trick and run away." I kept hoping she would send me a message telling me where we could meet secretly again.

As I got older, I began to take more notice of the boys in my class. I particularly liked one of them, a shy, tousle-haired, blond young boy who came to school in overalls. His parents owned one of the farms where we bought our produce, and I would see him working in the fields during the summer. After we had been in a few grades together we became friendlier. He wasn't much of a student, but he was the star of the baseball team and I was delighted when he offered to bring me a lemonade during the party held at the end of the school year. We sat sipping lemonade and talking until the party ended, when he offered to walk me home. As we set out together, some of the other children began to chant, "Jimmy is a Jew-lover! Jimmy is a Jew-lover!" I ran away, sobbing, "I'll go home by myself!"

Dad adapted to Schroon Lake as if he had been born there. Tall and muscular, with bronzed skin, high cheekbones, and hawk-like nose, he could easily have been mistaken for a member of the Indian tribes who came to town for their weekly supplies. He usually wore a heavy, red and black checked flannel shirt and dungarees, like most of the other men in town. Even in summer the mornings were cold, and none of us changed to lighter clothes until the sun had warmed us.

Dad made friends easily. He hired some of the local men to help him with his building projects and eventually constructed a colony of eight cottages for summer rental, increasing our income considerably. With an instinctive love of nature, he surrounded each cottage with flowering bushes and left most of the trees on the property untouched. He also expanded the main house, building bedrooms and a porch in back so that we didn't have to live in the attic. He built solidly, to last. The cottages and the main house are still standing today, over half a century later. But the people who eventually bought the property from us cut down the trees and bushes to make room for more buildings. The natural, attractive atmosphere that blended so well with the Adirondack landscape is gone, and when I visited Schroon Lake years later I could barely recognize the place.

But the town itself seemed as lovely as ever, with its one main street, and the bandstand in the park where a "concert" took place weekly when I was a child. The bandmaster, a rotund, gray-haired gentleman with a walrus moustache, wore a brilliant red uniform with gold epaulets and gold buttons. He played the tuba and his "oom-pah" dominated all the music. We also celebrated the Fourth of July in the park. The celebration would start with a parade through the town, proudly led by war veterans with their banners, followed by the school's marching band and the children, with American flags and red, white and blue streamers on their bicycles. The parade would end at the park, where a square dance and fireworks were held in the evening. We had a weekly square dance. I loved to listen to the sing-song chant of the caller and the country music. To this day, I love to square dance.

My father was well-respected in town, "even though he's a Jew." He was meticulously honest in all his business dealings, paid his bills promptly, and was admired for his independence and hard work in undertaking most of the projects on our land by himself. He became part of a group of cronies who paid him the ultimate compliment of inviting him to go deer hunting in the fall. He had purchased a rifle because we lived in a rather isolated area and he felt we needed protection from wild animals—both two-footed and four-footed. Since this was his first experience hunting deer, his friends positioned him along the trail so he would have the first shot. A young buck suddenly crashed through the forest only a short distance from where he was hiding. My father took one look at the animal's terrified eyes, raised his rifle—and fired directly up in the air. The deer bounded away, unhurt. His friends were disgusted. He admitted sheepishly, "I couldn't kill that animal."

He never went hunting again, but he taught my brothers and me how to handle a gun. We all became pretty good shots. As the kid sister, I had become quite competitive and was anxious to show my brothers that I could shoot as well as they could. Our favorite target was the brass knob on top of the huge flagpole my father had erected on the roof of the main house. When we hit it, the bullet would cause it to "ping" and we would count how many "pings" we got in ten shots. I was proud that I could more than hold my own. Looking back now, I realize that was not a safe activity and probably would be considered illegal, but that didn't occur to us then.

My parents and I stayed after the tourist season so that my father could make repairs and do more building. He filled in the marshy areas leading to the lake by trucking in loads of sand that he shoveled by hand. The sand came from a huge quarry in the heart of a forest that stretched up the mountain across the road from us. Completely friendless after Ellie's death, I created an imaginary life around that quarry. I discovered a secret hiding place where I loved to go and read undisturbed. My favorite books were adventure stories, like *Tarzan of the Apes*, by Edgar Rice Burroughs. The quarry became the elephants' graveyard that fascinated me in the Tarzan series. Later on I graduated to historical novels, like *Scaramouche*, by Raphael Sabatini. I discovered these books myself in the library. I had very little direction from teachers about reading material until I was in high school.

On my way up to the quarry, I would pass many wild blackberry and raspberry bushes and I would often fill a basket with ripe berries for my mother's famous fruit pies. One sunny day, as I was picking berries from a large bush that had grown taller than I was, I heard some rustling on the other side and assumed it was one of the numerous birds who also loved to eat the berries. As I rounded the bush, I came nose to nose with a large brown bear. I screamed and he howled and we took off in opposite directions as fast as we could run. I don't know who was the more terrified.

Without any playmates, I was left pretty much to my own resources. I loved to help my mother in the kitchen, inhaling the delicious aroma of fresh-baked pies, puddings, and cakes. When the restaurant became busy in the afternoon, I would be in the way and would wander off to find other ways of amusing myself. Some days I would go to the quarry to read, surrounded by the quiet and the fragrance of the piney woods. In the summer I would swim every day. I really can't remember an age when I couldn't swim. My brothers had a tradition of swimming across the lake—about three miles—at least once each year and I joined them as soon as my parents would permit it. My father would not allow us to take such a long swim without a boat to accompany us.

Another annual event that I shared with my brothers was a hike up Mt. Pharaoh, one of the high peaks in the Adirondacks, just across the lake from us. Mt. Pharaoh plays an important role in my memories of Schroon Lake. Many years later, before Al Schrager and I were married, he came to visit my family and we decided to climb to the top of the mountain. It was a beautiful, sunny day when we started but as we approached the summit the sky became black and it began to pour. We were in the midst of a violent thunderstorm and were completely exposed to the elements. I had often seen lightening strike the top of the mountain and we climbed rapidly to reach the shelter of the forest ranger's station above us. Exhausted, I realized I couldn't keep up with Al. I was panic-stricken and felt responsible for putting the man I loved in such peril. I collapsed against a rock, rain streaming down my face and gasped, "I can't go on. Just leave me here. Save yourself." Al looked at me with the quizzical expression he developed when quietly amused. He said, "Glor, if you would stop emoting and catch your breath, we'll be okay." And of course we were.

I smile as I think of these memories now, but the years in Schroon Lake were very lonely. Yet, in searching for diversions, I developed skills that otherwise I would not have. There was a riding stable close to our property and in exchange for doing some chores, the owners let me ride. There was one horse I particularly loved: a gentle mare who had a unique gait called single-foot. When we galloped, it was like being on a rocking chair. Years later, Al and I vacationed in Puerto Rico with our children and I asked the manager of the hotel's riding school if any of his horses had this gait. He said, "Down here, we call it Peso Fino. One of my horses has it, but I don't usually let guests ride him. If you think you can manage him, I'll let you try." He was a beautiful white stallion and the exhilaration of that early morning gallop along the beach was unforgettable. The children were anxious to see the horse and we agreed that they could take pictures when I rode him the next day. When I got into the saddle and the camera clicked, he reared straight up, pawing the air and snorting. I was able to hold my seat but the boys began to cry. Al roared, "Get down from there; you're the mother of children!" It was a long time before I rode again.

When we first moved to Schroon Lake, acid rain was not as much of a problem as it is now. The lake abounded with fish and I would spend hours fishing from one of the boats my father had built. I became expert in finding the good fishing spots. Late one afternoon a torrential downpour had ended, the sun had come out, and I thought it a particularly good time to fish. I headed for one of my favorite spots, some distance from the house and found that the fish, mostly rock bass and perch, were indeed biting furiously. I was so busy hauling them in, I didn't notice the dense fog rolling over the lake. It was growing dark, and my father came down to the lake with a lantern and shouted for me to come home but I couldn't hear him. Sound and light were muffled by the fog. Thoroughly alarmed, he ran back to the house for a huge frying pan, began banging it against a big rock near the lake while waving his lantern with his other hand and shouting himself hoarse. I still couldn't hear him but decided I had caught as many fish as we could possibly use and headed home. The fog was so dense I couldn't see the front of the boat, much less any landmarks but I knew the general direction to go. As I got closer, I could hear my father's shouts, the clamor of the frying pan and I could see the dim light of the lantern through the fog. Somewhat guiltily I called, "I'm coming."

As soon as I landed, I knew I was in big trouble. I had never seen my father so angry with me. I held up the huge string of fish, so heavy I could barely lift them and said," Dad, look how many fish I caught." He stopped his tirade in mid-sentence and grunted:" Don't ever do that to us again. You had us scared half to death."

I usually went to bed early, but occasionally I would go out to look at the millions of stars and try to identify constellations. There were nights when the aurora borealis shone with its ever-changing mystical light. I looked forward to the summer evening when the only movie in town, the Rialto, opened for the tourist season. It was opened only on weekends for two evening performances. The movie was changed weekly. Since my parents would not permit me to walk to the village alone after dark and since they could not close the business to take me to the movies, I was dependent on my brothers or on visitors if I wanted to see a show. One week a musical starring Nelson Eddy and Jeannette McDonald was playing. They were my favorite movie stars and my brothers were going to the movies that week with some visiting cousins. I asked to come along but they refused to take me. I can understand the reasons now: they were probably planning some amusement after the show that could not be shared with a pesky kid sister. I begged and pleaded and after my parents urged them, they reluctantly agreed. I ran happily to my room to get a sweater. When I came back, I found that they had driven off without me. I was overcome with grief and disappointment. To this day, I often harbor anxieties of being left behind. It may also be the reason why I am so meticulous about keeping promises, especially to children. And it probably was the start of my fierce determination to be independent and never have to ask anybody for anything.

CHAPTER THREE

The Horrors of the City

My parents would close the business in November after my father made repairs at the end of the tourist season and finished whatever new building he had planned. Our house did not have enough insulation to withstand the bitter winter cold. Since all tourist activity ceased during the winter so did all income. Although unemployment was still high, my father, with his metal-working skills, was usually able to find some part-time job in the city for the winter months.

October and November used to be moving time in the city when everybody seemed to switch to a different apartment. My parents had no difficulty in renting an apartment for the several winter months in Brooklyn. It was always different but always the same: a small, dark place, usually on the second or third floor of a dingy walk-up apartment house, where the hallways forever retained the stale, pungent odor of cooked cabbage and spiced meats and garlic.

My parents' personalities seemed to change drastically in the city. At Schroon Lake, my mother had become self-confident and articulate, a gracious hostess in her restaurant. During the winter, she was silent and withdrawn. She became quite deferential to my father's family, weighed down by the money we owed them. (We eventually repaid it all, with interest.) My aunt and my grandmother (my father's mother) treated my mother like a servant. She was expected to cook and serve at every social function. She never objected. I became increasingly resentful of this as I grew older. My mother wanted me to show similar deference not only to my aunt but also to her daughters. I refused. The idea of acting like a poor relation was insupportable. Both daughters, several years older than I, either ignored me or treated me with contempt.

My mother's relationship with her own family also changed. We were no longer part of that warm inner circle. There was still great affection between my mother and her four brothers but her sisters-in-law were cold and openly critical of the way we lived. She on her part resented their treatment of her mother. Before our move to Schroon Lake, my mother's parents had lived with us but now no one would take in my widowed grandmother. She had no income of her own (these were the days before Social Security) and she was totally dependent on her children. They placed her in a nursing home where she was miserable. She was a very intelligent woman, literate in both Russian and Yiddish and loved to read and discuss the day's events. The books she wanted and the people to talk to were no longer available to her. When we were in the city, we used to visit her often. I remember carrying on long conversations with her, she speaking Yiddish, I answering in English. We understood each other perfectly but neither could speak the other's native tongue.

My father underwent an even greater change in the city. He was cheerful and garrulous at Schroon Lake, drinking beer with his friends who came to the restaurant in the evening. He obviously enjoyed the hard manual work he did each day and he would seek advice from his friends concerning the plans he had for our property. He took great pride in its appearance and loved the outdoors. Once, when ill with a cough and fever, he said "Just let me get one sniff of that good mountain air and I'll be cured."

We left the city earlier than usual that spring, with patches of snow still on the ground. Dad drove the car for the eight-hour trip despite his illness. My mother was terrified for his health but she could not stop him. The mountain air cure apparently worked: within a day he was back to his old self.

Dad hated the winter months and became irritable and argumentative. His sister felt it was her prerogative to tell him how to run the business and he would explode with fury. She would scream back in Yiddish, "Dein Gelt geht in dr'erde" unaware that this was a double entendre. A familiar Yiddish curse is "Gehe in dr'erde!" which translated literally means "Go into the earth!" but whose actually meaning is "Drop dead!" So my aunt meant that my father was wasting, or destroying, his money, his "Gelt". She did not realize that the saying was true in a more literal sense. He was indeed plowing his money back into the earth, filling in marshland with truckloads of sand, transforming with his own hands an uninhabitable area into an attractive summer resort.

Our annual move to the city and back again made my schooling increasingly erratic. I would start each school year in the fall at Schroon Lake, transfer in the middle of the term to a school in the city, start the spring term there, and transfer in the middle of that term back to Schroon Lake where I would finish the school year. Since the apartments my parents rented were in different school districts each year, I attended many different schools. School districting was confusing and I would often have to walk considerable distances to the assigned school.

Although I tried to make friends with the children in my class, I could not. They would laugh and mimic the strange new girl. Unwittingly I had acquired some speech patterns and mannerisms from Schroon Lake. For example, the people there would say "ayah" instead of "yes" and speak in a slow drawl, much different from the rapid-fire city speech. I hated to be laughed at and became a tight-lipped loner. As alien as I felt in Schroon Lake, I felt even more so in these strange, inhospitable urban surroundings.

I was becoming a tall, gangly, unattractive adolescent with curly black hair that was thick and unruly. I was not a happy child and had developed a perpetually anxious look, due in part to nearsightedness, unrecognized for many years. As I grew older, the constant transferring from one school to another became increasingly difficult. I began to have nightmares about taking exams for which I was totally unprepared, on material I had never learned. Many people have similar dreams but mine were based on reality.

I disliked the city, its schools and its teachers. Discipline was strict and the method of teaching seemed to be by instilling fear. We had to wear uniforms—the girls in white middy blouses with a navy tie and a navy pleated skirt. My parents could only afford to buy me one set and every night my mother would launder the blouse so it would be clean and starched for the next day. We had to line up in the school yard to have our attendance taken and wait there until the bell rang to allow us in. This occurred in all kinds of winter weather and we girls, with our short coats and ankle socks, were often shivering with the cold by the time we could enter the building.

A crisis was reached when I was in junior high in the city, about 1936, and had a teacher, Miss Mitchell, whom I feared and disliked. All the female teachers were unmarried. Marriage disqualified them from employment and if the authorities found out that they had secretly married, their jobs were instantly terminated. Miss Mitchell never smiled and often humiliated the children with remarks about dirty or bitten fingernails and untidy hair. In teaching us about immigration to this country, she said in her high screechy voice that grated on my nerves like chalk across a blackboard, "The desirable people have come to our country from England, Scotland and northern Europe but they were followed by undesirables from Eastern Europe and Italy."

I was becoming increasingly ashamed of my origins. Moe, now in his mid-twenties, sat down to talk to me. It was the first time I understood what the word "bigot" meant. Moe told me how proud I should be of our people. They had made wonderful contributions to this country. He told me about Einstein. "And the governor of New York State, Herbert Lehman, is a Jew," he said. "The mayor of our city, Fiorello LaGuardia, is Italian. Ask your teacher if she thinks they are undesirable." Of course I was too afraid to challenge Miss Mitchell in any way, but I felt better about myself.

One day Miss Mitchell announced that we were going to have a surprise quiz. "I want to be sure you've all been doing your work at home," she said. It was based on material from the beginning of the term, when I had not yet joined the class. No one did very well and she vented her anger by having all the children who had failed stand and publicly announce their grade. She then proceeded to humiliate each in turn. I knew that I would be the last since mine was by far the lowest grade. I had points taken off for incorrect guesses. As I stood waiting my turn, fearful and ashamed, I had one of my very rare flashes of temper. I screamed, "I hate you, I hate you! I'm never coming back to this stupid school again!" I rushed out of the class and ran home sobbing.

My parents were horrified, expecting the truant officer to come after our family. Moe again took matters in hand. He went to see the school's principal the next day. Together, they coaxed me to return. To my surprise, I now found that Miss Mitchell seemed more afraid of me than I was of her. Looking back, it may be why I never considered becoming a teacher when I grew up. Except for my elementary school teacher in Schroon Lake, I never liked any teacher until I was in high school. I noted that, though they could bully the children, the teachers could be easily intimidated by their superiors. They were mostly women, their superiors—the principals and superintendents—mostly men. My teachers were not role models to instill feelings of independence and self-respect.

The incident in junior high convinced my parents that the constant transfer to different schools was not a good idea. Since I was about to start high school and they could not provide the continuity of a permanent home in the city, I was sent to live with my aunt at the beginning of the school year until my parents would return to the city for the winter months. My aunt was the matriarch of the family who had loaned my father the money to buy our property at Schroon Lake. She was a heavy woman with jet black hair and unsmiling dark eyes. Her swarthy complexion resembled my father's. Married to a pharmacist, her family was by far the most prosperous of all our relatives. They lived in one of two very comfortable adjoining homes in Brooklyn, sharing a common driveway. The houses were of yellow stucco and had many windows. They were both furnished in a Victorian way, the parlors crowded with overstuffed furniture and many little tables laden with family pictures and knickknacks. My father's youngest brother, a dentist, and his family lived in the house next door.

My aunt accepted my presence with poor grace. She wanted me to live in the attic, a large gloomy place that ran the length of the house above the second floor where the family slept. One end of the attic was occupied by an older brother who was demented. A stooped, gray-haired man who walked with a strange lope, he had apparently been normal until drafted into the Czar's army. He had been beaten unmercifully many times, had become mentally unstable, and was sent home. His wife and children had left him when he emigrated to the U.S. with my aunt and her family. He wandered the streets each day talking to himself and would occasionally have wild rages, running around the house with a knife. But he never harmed anyone. I was terrified of him even though he completely ignored me. Still, I stubbornly refused to live in the attic and would creep down to sleep in my oldest cousin's empty bed when she left for college. My aunt didn't like the idea but after a while she gave up trying to stop me. That didn't keep her from expressing her displeasure at my presence, particularly when she talked to other members of the family.

Our extended family had a Cousins' Club that met monthly. Besides being a social gathering, dues were collected for various charities and worthy causes. After the business meeting, the men would play cards and smoke cigars. I loved the aroma of the cigars, fruity and pleasant. That and the soft laughter and murmur of voices made the house seem cozy and secure. It was good to have a sense of belonging. I would play with my cousins and the women would drink tea and chat.

At one of these meetings I heard my aunt complaining about the difficulty of having me live with her. "She is not a pleasant child—I've even caught her stealing!"

My mother's niece, Leah, was a married woman noted for her sharp tongue. She was tall and gaunt and fiercely loyal to my mother. "I can't believe a child of this family would steal," she said. "Tell me, what has she taken?"

"She sneaks lumps of sugar from the sugar bowl into her pocket every morning on the way to school."

"You call that stealing?" shrieked Leah. "You should be ashamed of yourself!"

I did indeed sneak lumps of sugar into my pocket on the way to school. Each day I would pass a milk wagon drawn by a scrawny old horse. I looked forward to feeding him the sugar. It got to the point where he would recognize my footsteps, whinny softly as I approached, and nuzzle me after he had his treat. I would kiss him on the nose. It was the only affection I gave or received during my stay at my aunt's house.

I was often hungry. I did not dare go to the refrigerator after the sugar lump episode, and no one made me lunch to take to school. My parents had given me some money but I did not have enough to buy lunch each day. I had become close friends with a girl named Nina in my French class and we loved to spend our free time talking French and going to museums to see the French Impressionist paintings. Her mother, a warm, caring woman, always insisted that I had a "snack" when I came to visit. When she discovered I did not eat lunch, she packed an extra sandwich for me in Nina's lunch bag. I wanted to show my appreciation and finally had an inspired thought. I had been active on several athletic teams and had won some swimming meets. I also had been elected secretary of the G.O., the General Organization that ran the student government. And I had become an editor of the school newspaper. Because of these activities, I had acquired a bunch of school athletic letters and service pins. I gave some of them to Nina. Her mother laughed and shook her head. "Things like that have to be earned and not given away as gifts."

"But Nina did earn them," I insisted.

I wasn't the only one who knew the hunger of an unwanted guest. My brothers had also "spent time" at my aunt's house when they were in college. And they couldn't creep down to our cousins' beds, but had to live in the attic. We laughed about it years later. Moe said he existed on American cheese. He never could abide the taste of American cheese after that. He used to raid the refrigerator, often caught by my paternal grandmother. She would take a broomstick to chase him away. She was a stooped, scowling, bitter woman whose gray hair was gathered into a bun that she wore at the top of her head. She, like my aunt, never showed me or my brothers any affection.

She was very respectful towards my aunt's husband, the pharmacist, who was considered part of the Russian intelligentsia. A short, florid man with a pince-nez, he always wore a three-piece blue serge suit, with a watch in his vest pocket. The watch was attached to a gold chain that swooped across his expansive belly to be attached to the vest on the other side. Hanging from the chain was a key from the Rotary Club which he rubbed between his fingers as he pontificated on world events at the dinner table. He would often pace the floor, arms folded behind his back, shaking his balding head and making philosophical remarks, like a character in a Chekov play. Most of these remarks were in Russian, but occasionally he would lapse into a mixture of Hebrew and Yiddish. The one I remember best is "Rabboinische Olim! Der Olim ist ein Golem!" ("Master of the Universe! The World has Gone Mad!") I could understand how he felt after listening to the radio, with Hitler screaming his hatred and Britain's Prime Minister Chamberlain appeasing him, promising us "peace in our time."

My grandmother felt that my brothers and I, children of an arbeitermensch (workingman) had no right to an education. When she found out that Moe, during his senior year at college, was helping his chemistry professor with some research, she scolded, "He should be out making money to support his parents! He could be driving a taxi in his spare time!" She was scarcely mollified when he was appointed an instructor in chemistry at Brooklyn College shortly after he graduated and was able to marry and set up a home independently.

My parents' income from Schroon Lake was limited to the summer season but one winter they were offered jobs in a hotel in Florida, run by friends. Since it was difficult to stretch the income from the summer months to last all year, they decided to accept. It meant that I would be living in my aunt's house without seeing them for almost six months. I missed them terribly. When Christmas came, my aunt and her family and my uncle's family next door all went to Florida to visit them. My parents could not afford to pay for my trip, and my relatives were unwilling to do so, and I was left behind, with an unloving grandmother and a demented uncle.

Life has a way of taking care of these matters. Years later, during my fellowship at New York Hospital, my aunt came to visit at my parents' house. She appeared to acknowledge for the first time that I was an adult and perhaps even a doctor. She tried to hide her anxiety. "I found a lump in my breast, and I went to see our family doctor. He told me he was one hundred percent sure I had nothing to worry about."

I said, "I don't know how he can be so certain without a biopsy. Look, I'm working now just across the street from Memorial Sloan-Kettering. They have some of the most famous breast specialists in the world. If you like, I'll make an appointment for you to be seen there."

She reluctantly agreed. The mass was malignant, and she had a radical mastectomy. There was a shortage of private nurses and so I stayed at her bedside for 48 hours, until they could find one. When she was discharged from the hospital, she wrote out a check for my services. I refused to take it. "I hope this partially repays you for all your sacrifices when I was a little girl." I don't think she got the irony of my remark.

Her gratitude did not last long. She became increasingly resentful of the bills for her follow-up visits. She decided that she hadn't had cancer after all since she was still alive and well several years later. She was sure it was all a plot to extort money from her and I was involved. Her daughter developed a mass in her breast a short time later and decided she would not be fooled by doctors as her mother had been. She did not seek medical care until the spreading cancer made the diagnosis self-evident. When she finally went to a doctor, he was furious because of the neglect which had caused the disease to be so far advanced. His lack of sympathy increased their family's dislike of the medical profession. She died a short time later. My aunt lived into old age.

I felt guilty because, unlike the rest of the family, I could never truly mourn my cousin's death. When I had lived in their house she had subjected me to many petty humiliations. Since we couldn't afford new clothes, I had to wear her cast-off belongings. These were never handed down with any grace or sensitivity, but just thrown in my general direction. She was several years ahead of me in the same high school. She never showed any interest in my activities or offered companionship because I was alone. She took pleasure in embarrassing me. The only way I could retaliate was by trying to best her scholastically in every way I could. She was proud of being a reporter on the school newspaper. I became editor-in-chief. She had received some honors at graduation. I became valedictorian, with a larger number of honors.

After graduation, both she and her older sister went to Smith College, one of the most prestigious women's colleges in the country. I was determined to go there, too. But here I could not compete because my parents could not afford it. Although I was offered a partial scholarship, the expenses were still overwhelming. Sobbing dramatically, I threw my acceptance into the kitchen stove at Schroon Lake and knew that the only college open to me was one of the tuition-free city colleges. It was probably one of the luckiest things that ever happened to me.

CHAPTER FOUR

The Spanish Civil War and WW II

M y years in high school (1937-1941) partially coincided with the Spanish Civil War (1936-1939). My sympathies were with the Loyalists and I decided to go to Washington for a student rally on their behalf. The rally was sponsored by the American Student Union (the ASU) and although I was not a member, I joined to be eligible to ride in their buses. I had never been active politically and that rally made a lasting impression. The meeting was run by Joe Lash, president of the ASU, who later became a close friend of Eleanor Roosevelt. Mrs. Roosevelt spoke and also attended several of our sessions. I remember her sitting a few rows in front of me, quietly knitting.

It was probably her influence that made FDR agree to address us on the White House lawn. We stood in the pouring rain, shouting, "Lift the Embargo on Loyalist Spain!" We didn't have to stand there long. FDR's message was brief. He scolded us for having the temerity to try to influence the decisions of our elders. He then ordered us, in avuncular fashion, to disperse immediately and get into some dry clothes. "That is," he added with an attempt at jocularity, "if you *have* dry clothes." I was angry and ashamed. My parents worshipped FDR, and although I had the impression that their god had feet of clay, I felt I had disgraced them.

The majority of students in the ASU had no political affiliations but there was a core that belonged to the Young Communist League, the YCL. After the rally, members of the YCL urged me to join. I declined. There was something unthinking about the way they always adhered to the party line. This became particularly evident after Stalin signed a nonaggression pact with Hitler. They kept repeating as if by rote the party's slogan, "Capitalism is just as bad as Nazism." I was disgusted because I knew that many were intelligent people who certainly had the capacity to think independently. It was bewildering to me that they could suspend their own judgement to follow leaders whose agenda was suspect.

During these high-school years, when I lived with my aunt, I developed a Cinderella complex and kept hoping for a fairy godmother who would rescue me from my life of poverty and loneliness. I did not expect that the "fairy godmother" would appear in the form of a bristling, mustached terror of a professor at Brooklyn College, who would change my whole life.

I entered college in September, 1941. We were not yet in World War II, although our sympathies were strongly with the British and FDR had instituted his Lend Lease program, shipping supplies to England. Germany had overrun most of Europe but there was still a very vocal, isolationist group in the United States, the "America First" movement. A portion of that group was openly sympathetic with Hitler and claimed that the world could be very comfortably divided between two superpowers—The United States and Germany. Two of the most influential members of that group were Joseph P. Kennedy, our ambassador to England, and Charles Lindberg, our American hero, who had flown across the Atlantic successfully in a small plane. Both claimed that it was the Jews who were responsible for pushing us toward a war that was none of our business.

That group became less vocal after December 7, 1941, when the Japanese bombed Pearl Harbor. I will never forget that day, a Sunday. I was reading quietly, waiting to sit down to dinner with my parents. Their finances had improved and they were able to rent a pleasant apartment full-time in the city. Moe had recently married and he and his wife, Sylvia Bregman, had been invited to join us for dinner. (My brother Milton was in the army and was stationed at Fort Belvoir, in Virginia.) The radio was tuned to WQXR. Suddenly a Mozart symphony was interrupted by the shocking news that we had been attacked. We were told that FDR would address the nation the next day, Monday, at noon.

Morning classes at college that Monday were quite disorganized with the war on everyone's lips. At noon the entire college gathered outside in the quadrangle to hear FDR, his voice booming over the loud-speakers, "On December 7, a day that will live in infamy . . . ."

We dispersed quietly after his talk. I went to my next class in modern dance in the gym, and changed into shorts and a sleeveless gym shirt. We had barely begun the class when air raid sirens began to wail. Several unidentified planes had been sighted approaching New York.

We were told to evacuate the building immediately without waiting to dress or get our outer garments. All was confusion. December weather is not exactly conducive to wearing a scanty gym uniform outdoors and we were hopping around to keep warm. We begged to be allowed inside for just a moment to get our coats, but the building was locked. After a time, with no one apparently in charge I decided, "This is ridiculous. I'm not going to waste my energy jumping up and down. I'm going home." We lived about three miles from the college, and the buses or trolleys that I usually took were not running. I set off at a brisk trot, passing confused groups of people who had also been ordered to evacuate their buildings. They were standing in the street, many staring with amazement at the young girl jogging by in gym shorts. The "all clear" sounded just about the time I reached home. It had been a false alarm.

It took a while for this country to get an effective air-raid service organized with designated shelters. I volunteered to be an air-raid warden for my block. Women were just beginning to be accepted for that kind of duty and I was very proud of my arm-band and helmet. We were all fingerprinted by the FBI. I wonder if they still have my prints on file.

It is hard to remember all the accommodations we had to make because of the war. We had rationing, with a certain number of stamps for various products. I remember pooling stamps with other members of the family so we had enough eggs and sugar to bake a cake for Passover. There was a strict blackout and we had dark shades to cover our windows at night. Air-raid wardens took turns patrolling the street to make sure no light leaked through. Huge beams raked the sky in search of enemy aircraft. Broadway and the surrounding theater area were dark. Cars had the upper halves of their curved headlights painted black so that the only light was directed downwards. A popular song was the sentimental ballad, "When the Lights Go On Again, All Over the World."

Although the continental U.S. was never attacked, we felt the immediacy of the war through newspaper accounts, the radio, and newsreels. I remember Edward R. Murrow broadcasting from London, the sounds of bombs in the background. Newsreels were shown in every movie theater, updated weekly. We followed the bombing of Britain, the blitzkrieg, and saw the damage and the suffering. We saw Hitler ranting before massed crowds shouting, "Seig Heil!" with arms extended in the Nazi salute. We saw him dancing a jig when Paris fell. We saw Mussolini, his jaw jutting forward, exhorting the Italian people. There was no TV but I doubt that our involvement was any less because we didn't have these scenes in our living room each day.

I had no idea how deeply I was affected. Years later, after we were married, Al and I were touring Europe and stopped for several days in Vienna. We were having a delightful time until one day we were crossing the Heldenplatz on our way to see the Lippenzaner stallions perform in the Spanish Riding School. The Heldenplatz is a huge open plaza with equestrian statues at one end and a ring of palaces and public buildings at the other. We were halfway across the plaza when I experienced the only panic attack I've ever had in my life. I felt exposed and trapped. Heart beating wildly, I raced for the shelter of the buildings and stood there trembling. Al, deeply concerned, ran after and held me, asking what was wrong. I gasped, pointing to one of the balconies of a building facing the plaza, "Hitler was there. I could feel it. He stood on that balcony and the entire Heldenplatz was filled with storm troopers."

As soon as I regained my composure we continued to the Riding School, located in one of the palaces. A man was sitting at a large desk collecting tickets. Al, who could speak fluent German, asked with a charming smile, "Did Hitler ever speak in the Heldenplatz.?"

"Ja," said the man proudly, and pulled from one of the desk drawers an album with newspaper clippings. "I don't show this to many tourists," he confided. One of the clippings had a picture of Hitler standing on a balcony hung with swastikas, addressing German soldiers in the Heldenplatz. It was just as I had described it. My only explanation was that I must have seen it in a newsreel during those war years and it had made a lasting impression on my subconscious.

The rest of my first year of college passed quickly, with my increasing disinterest in the courses I was taking. The war dominated all our thoughts. In addition to my history courses, I took a dance class, a writing seminar, and an art course in fashion design. Ever since my experience wearing my cousin's castoff clothes I had developed an obsession about dressing well, and enjoyed sketching original designs. Unfortunately, wartime was not a time to indulge in such fantasies. Rationing was strict and clothing was practical and unattractive. Our supply of glamorous silk stockings had been cut off due to the war with Japan and nylons had just been invented. They were scarce and very expensive. We wore thick lisle stockings that would have made even a lovely dress look unattractive. The only women who wore pants, mostly men's overalls that fit the female figure badly, were factory and farm workers. I often wore men's jeans, called dungarees or Levi's, bought in the general store in Schroon Lake, but I never wore them in the city, and never to school. I don't recall anyone making pants for women—except for Hollywood stars like Marlene Dietrich and Katherine Hepburn.

My other courses seemed to have as little relevance as my art class. In choosing a schedule for my second year, I decided to take some science courses. I was disconcerted that my biology course was being taught by a holy terror named Professor Alexander Novikoff. I was particularly upset because I knew that Dr. Novikoff was a good friend of Moe and with no science background I feared I would be an embarrassment to my brother. What a relief to discover I could do well!

The weekend after Novikoff urged me to apply to medical school I spoke with my parents about my new ambition. The response was typical of what was to become the struggle of the next few years. The men in my life encouraged me, the women did not. My father, after his initial astonishment, said he would find ways of financing my education despite difficult economic circumstances. My mother was horrified. The idea of her daughter messing around with unpleasant, unwomanly things and ending up an old maid was quite devastating to her.

She had ample support from the extended family—my aunts, uncles, cousins—all of whom thought the scatterbrained whims of a thoughtless adolescent (and a girl!) should be ignored. Several took me aside to give me private lectures on the selfishness of even thinking to put that kind of strain on my family's limited resources.

There were many heated family conferences. The decisive voice was again that of my brother, Moe. As a teacher at Brooklyn College, he had a lot of influence with the family. "It won't be easy for a woman to get into medical school," he said. "Still, if she wants to try, she should. Women are less than 4 % of admissions and there are quotas for Jews in all the medical schools. So a Jewish woman from Brooklyn College hasn't got much chance. Glor, good luck, but don't be disappointed if it doesn't work out."

My first step was to see my faculty advisor. She was supposed to help us with career planning. "Who do you think you are?" she sneered. "Just because you've gotten some good grades, do you think you can compete with men for admission to medical school? Forget it. Now if you're interested in nursing . . ." I thanked her and left.

I sent away for applications to medical school and soon realized that I lacked most of the science requirements for admission. I spent the next year in a heavily-weighted program of physics, chemistry and biology courses. By the following June I had completed all necessary courses except for the second semester of organic chemistry. Because of wartime needs, schools were accepting students at the end of three years of college and I decided to apply for early admission.

I thought my best chance was at the Woman's Medical College of Pennsylvania, where male competition for admission would not be a problem. They accepted me with the proviso that I complete all requirements by the following September. This was June and I still hadn't taken the second half of organic chemistry. Looking around desperately for a college that was offering Organic II during the summer, I found that City College uptown was the only such institution in the metropolitan area. But City College at that time was all male. No women could apply.

Taking my provisional letter of acceptance with me, I made an appointment to see the Dean. After some hesitation he said, "Well, it's only a summer course. It's not as if you were applying to the college itself. I guess we can arrange it." And so for the rest of the summer I traveled daily from Brooklyn to upper Manhattan, a subway trip of almost two hours each way, in the sweltering New York heat. When I got to class we had to do steam distillations. The labs were not airconditioned and the temperature rose to over 100 degrees Fahrenheit. The men all stripped to the waist and urged me to do the same. I was tempted but didn't comply.

Milton (Mickey) had finished his basic training in the army and was being sent overseas. He had two weeks' leave before departure and planned to spend them at Schroon Lake with my parents. Those two weeks coincided with the last two weeks of my summer course. I explained the problem to my lab instructor, requesting permission to take the final examination two weeks early. He consented and so I cut my brief summer review of Organic II even shorter. Moe also came to visit for a short time before Mickey shipped out. Together we climbed Mt. Pharoah. Mickey, in superb physical shape after finishing basic training, set the pace up the mountain while Moe and I eyed each other surreptitiously, neither of us willing to be the one to suggest the usual rest stops. We reached the summit in record time. Moe and I threw ourselves on the ground, gasping and wheezing. Mickey stared at us in amazement and alarm and said apologetically, "Gee, guys, why didn't you tell me you had to rest?" We grinned, admitting that good ol' sibling rivalry had been at work.

Someone agreed to take a picture of the three of us. It is one of my favorites. Three young people, our hair blowing in the wind, sitting on the rocky summit, glorying in the beautiful weather and the view and enjoying our own health and vigor and companionship. This would be our last picture together before embarking on the grim business of adulthood.

CLIMBING MT. PHARAOH

Mickey, Moe and Me On Our Last Climb Together, 1944

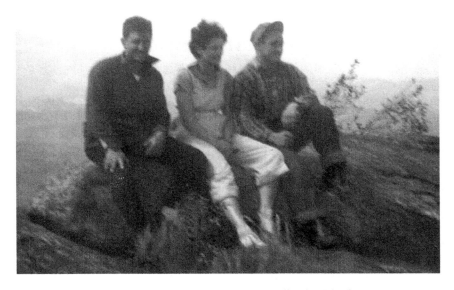

Al Schrager On His First Climb, 1948

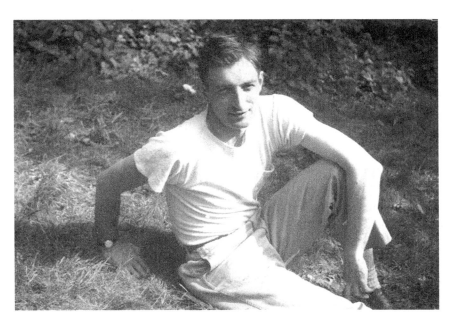

CHAPTER FIVE

Medical School

I passed my summer course in Organic Chemistry without difficulty although my grade went down a notch because I had elected to take the final exam two weeks early. Woman's Medical College accepted me and in September of 1944 I left for Philadelphia. My uncle Herschel, a tailor, had made me a new suit for the occasion. He had sewn it lovingly out of heavy blue gabardine, cut in a severe mannish style. It was not very flattering but it was extremely durable and lasted me for years. I departed wearing my new suit and dragging my microscope. The school didn't supply such equipment during the war years. An agency rented them at a price, but my parents were able to buy a used one through Moe. They felt it would be cheaper in the long run and an investment in the future. I had very little other luggage.

I had commuted to college from my parents' apartment and assumed there would be dormitories or other facilities to which I would be assigned—a very false assumption. We were supposed to make our own arrangements for room and board but no one had told me. And so on the day of admission I found myself homeless, forlorn and terribly homesick. Most of the women in the entering class were much older than I and formed tight little groups from which I felt excluded. Many had known each other from previous occupations as nurses, social workers or missionaries, and also knew women in the upper classes who had helped them find living quarters. I felt completely lost in the hubbub of registration.

"I don't have a Philadelphia address" I said meekly. "I thought I would be living in a dormitory."

The registrar looked at me severely. "This is a graduate school, not an undergraduate college. We expect our students to have the maturity and responsibility to make their own living arrangements."

I was overcome by the fear that she thought me unfit for this school but said in a falsely confident voice, "Oh, I'll find a place to stay before the day is out."

I felt physically ill. It was not all due to the panic of homelessness. Typhoid fever was still endemic in Philadelphia and all students got a typhoid shot the first day of each school year. The vaccine was not as purified as it is now and the shot was painful. We all ran fevers for a day or so.

Students rented apartments or boarded with families in the surrounding neighborhood of East Falls and of course all the desirable spots had been taken. I found a boarding house in Germantown, a twenty-minute trolley car ride from the school. I boarded with the Hancocks, the husband a descendant of John Hancock. Mr. Hancock and his wife, who were childless, had fallen on hard times and had converted their beautiful old house to take in boarders. They were an elderly couple who retained a great sense of dignity despite their reduced financial circumstances. Mr. Hancock towered over his wife, a thin, fragile woman who always had a shawl wrapped around her as if perpetually cold. Her wrinkled face bore the look of many hardships and disappointments but she was proud to announce to all potential boarders that she still maintained her membership in the Daughters of the American Revolution (the DAR). Mr. Hancock, obese, with a red bulbous nose that betrayed a fondness for the bottle, showed me around the house. There was a musty smell of old furniture, heavy curtains and unopened books in the front parlor. A large bookcase with locked glass doors was filled with magnificent antiques from colonial times. "That silver serving piece was made by Paul Revere," Mr. Hancock said proudly. "It's been in my family since the Revolution. And that document came from Ben Franklin's printing press. I wouldn't part with any of these things for the world."

The parlor was crowded with furniture. Next to several stiff upholstered chairs were small carved wood tables on which stood faded photographs in silver frames. Old lamps with fringed silken shades did little to dispel the darkness of the room. The huge overstuffed sofa was covered with a faded blue and ivory brocade, frayed at the edges. Signs of wear on the arms and back were partially hidden by ivory-colored lace antimacassars. The sofa's heavy legs, of dark wood, were carved like lion's claws. A bay window, heavily curtained, admitted very little light in the room. It faced the narrow street which was still paved with cobblestones and lit by gas lamps.

Mr. Hancock showed me the vacant bedroom on the second floor. It was fairly large, with two windows that admitted more light than any of the rooms below. It was furnished with twin beds covered by white candlewick spreads, a large wardrobe for clothes, a desk, a small table and a sink with small mirror above it. There were no closets. The bathroom was down the hall, shared by boarders who occupied the three other bedrooms. I said instantly, "I'll take it!"

The other boarders were a diverse group of people. One was a soldier from a nearby army camp who was having an affair with an officer's wife. This was their place of assignation. One night we were awakened by the sound of pistol shots, screams and curses. The enraged husband had traced them and found them in flagrante delicto. The lady fled down the fire escape. The soldier was carted off by police ambulance. I never learned what happened to the three of them.

The day after I arrived, I discovered a student who was registering late and had been as negligent as I in planning for room and board. She was standing with her luggage outside the Dean's office when I went there to give them my new Philadelphia address. I said, "Hi. Do you have a place to live?" She shook her head disconsolately and I asked, "Would you like to room with me?" She enthusiastically agreed. Her name was Eva Reich and she became my only close friend in medical school. She was a cheerful, buxom young woman, the daughter of Dr. Wilhelm Reich, a Viennese psychiatrist. Eva spoke a heavily-accented English and, when excited, reverted to her native German. Some of her colloquialisms sent me into fits of laughter.

Wilhelm Reich had been Freud's heir apparent until he began writing about the function of the orgasm. This scandalized Freud's basically Victorian sensibilities, and the two psychiatrists became estranged. Still, Eva had many pleasant memories of Freud, whom she regarded as a surrogate grandfather. She remembered Freud bouncing her on his knee and had pictures of them together. The theories of Dr. Reich, involving his claims that he had isolated a specific life force which he called "orgone," were very popular in this country. He claimed this force could be accumulated in a large box, the orgone box. His patients would sit in the box, the size of a telephone booth, to benefit from its effects. Occasionally it affected them so much that they let forth a "primal scream" which was supposed to be helpful to their psyches. Eva was greatly influenced by her father and tried to get me to accept his theories. I listened politely although they seemed like pseudo-science to me.

One day an orgone box arrived at our boarding house. Dr. Reich had sent it to his daughter with an affectionate note: "I'm sure this will help you with your studies." It was enormous and very heavy and Mr. Hancock was ready to evict us. We had to pool our resources to hire someone to drag it up the stairs to our room on the second floor, removing the wardrobe so it would fit. From that day on, all our clothes and books were stored in the orgone box.

Settled at last, Eva and I could turn our attention to our studies. Our first year curriculum was quite daunting: anatomy, pathology, biochemistry, physiology, bacteriology, and some minor subjects I have forgotten. We received quite a lecture about respect for the human body before we were assigned to our cadavers. These were bodies that had been unclaimed when they died. I think we all had strong emotions about this rite of initiation. Many of the students crossed themselves. Some became faint and broke into a cold sweat. I remember feelings of nausea. I could not think of eating even after the class ended. My lack of appetite was not just psychological. The cadavers were preserved in formaldehyde which gave off a strong, pervasive, unforgettable odor that was very unpleasant. It clung to our clothes and to our bodies. Neither showers nor laundering could erase that smell.

As with everything else, you learn to adapt, particularly when you realize how much there is to learn. Before long we were deeply involved in our dissections and thought less about the origins of the inanimate objects on the tables in front of us. Four students were assigned to each cadaver. We were very dependent on each other. If one messed up her dissection the others couldn't follow the course of the nerve or blood vessel or other structure through that destroyed area. Every week we would have a "practical." Lab assistants would tie little red strings around various structures after we had finished class for the day, and the next day we would have to go from one body to the next, identifying these structures and explaining their functions. These practical exams were considered of greater importance than the less frequent written exams.

As I made the rounds of my first practical, I was startled to discover that I was colorblind! I couldn't see the red strings around some of the structures I had to identify. It was difficult to convince the faculty of my disability; it is extremely rare in women. They insisted I take Ishihara's test for colorblindness and stared incredulously at the results. I had never realized it before because actually I could see most colors quite well. I just saw them differently. The difficulty occurred when I had to look at tiny spots of color like the little red strings, or color that was a distance away like red chalk on a blackboard, or pale pastels. This also became a problem in bacteriology. Bacteria, on staining, were either Gram positive (blue) or Gram negative (red). I had to strain to identify the Gram negatives, but it's interesting how one adapts. What I couldn't make out by color, I learned to identify by shape or differences in shade.

I was twenty years old, but I had little knowledge of sex until that anatomy lab. Sex education in public schools was unheard of and girls particularly were "sheltered" until the ritual of a private talk with Mother before marriage. The importance of virginity was unquestioned and never discussed. I knew little about sexual anatomy but was soon enlightened. We had both male and female cadavers, usually placed alternately, so we could look at our neighbor's dissection and observe the anatomic differences in both sexes and discuss methods of coitus and reproduction.

Examinations in all subjects were frequent and intensive. Many students studied in groups but I felt more comfortable studying alone. That had been my method through all my previous schooling and it was difficult to change habits. Besides, an element of panic bordering on hysteria would often enter the groups. There was so much to learn and much of it was rote memory. Hearing a partner confuse different names, structures and functions only disturbed one's own learning process and I found I could do better by handling it myself. We knew that about a third of the class would flunk out at the end of the freshman year. This was not unique to Woman's Med. Many other schools, on the first day's orientation, would include the phrase: "Look to the right of you and the left of you. One of you will not be here next year." Little was done to relieve the stress.

Probably my most effective studying was done in the Wissahickon, a huge nature reserve just a few blocks from the college. I found a quiet, secluded spot that brought back memories of my refuge in the quarry at Schroon Lake. It afforded me the tranquility I badly needed. Whenever the weather permitted, I would take books and paper and trudge off to my hideaway. I found that I could learn best by writing down the required material and organizing it into lists, by structure or function. Of course we all used the time-honored devices, like remembering the cranial nerves by the mnemonic, "On Old Olympus Topmost Top, A Finn and German Viewed A Hop." Male medical students had a more obscene version, but this is the one we used. When my brain felt totally saturated, unable to retain one more fact, I would hike along one of the many trails that ran through the Wissahickon that stretched for miles. Refreshed, it was possible to return to my studies.

Probably the thing I despised most was the bone box. Each of us was given a large wooden box containing representative bones of the human skeleton. We wouldn't get an entire skeleton but just the bones of one arm, one leg, etc. The bones had various protuberances which occur naturally. Muscles or tendons are attached to bone in this manner. We had to learn the origins and insertions of all the different structures that attached to these varied bony protuberances. It was a discouraging task and I often became exasperated. I was not alone. During that year, a student at one of the other medical schools threw the contents of his bone box into the Schuylkill River. It took a while for the police to figure out the mystery of the dismembered corpse.

When the winter holidays came, I didn't have the train fare to go home. My parents offered to send me more money but I refused. They were having a hard enough time meeting my basic expenses. I told them it would be better if I stayed in Philadelphia studying for the exams that were to start the day after vacation. This was actually the truth. My brief exposure to the sciences in college put me at a disadvantage with the other students who had much stronger backgrounds. I was having a difficult time.

Late one afternoon I came back to the Hancocks' after spending the day in the school's laboratories and library. The house was eerily quiet. All the boarders were away for the holiday. Mrs. Hancock had taken a position as headmistress in a private girls' school and was rarely home. Still, I could usually hear Mr. Hancock puttering around. I called his name but got no response. Suddenly, I saw him lying inert on the floor in the front parlor. I knelt beside him and realized he had had a massive stroke. He was paralyzed but conscious, his features distorted. He was able to open one eye and muttered something incoherent. Somewhat incoherent myself, I stuttered, "Don't worry, Mr. Hancock. I'll get help."

There was no 911 in those days. Emergency Medical Services and Rescue Squads did not exist. I called the college hospital and learned that they did not have an ambulance service. They suggested that I call a private ambulance company. I was reluctant to do this, since neither the Hancocks nor I had any money. I looked frantically for Mrs. Hancock's phone number at work and for the name and number of their private doctor but could find neither. In desperation I called a student in her senior year with whom I had become friendly. She hurried over with her medical bag, examined him, and then suggested that we move him to a more comfortable spot on the sofa, where we could cover him with a blanket. The floor was very cold and his hands were like ice. He was a heavy man and pull and tug as we tried, we couldn't budge him. He opened his eye and glared at us with fury and contempt as we stood dithering over him, trying to decide what to do next. He managed to spit out one word: "Doctors!"

We finally called the city hospital, Philadelphia General, and they sent an ambulance that took him to a charity ward. He died there three days later. Mrs. Hancock put the house and its contents up for sale. All the precious antiques and documents were auctioned off. I was eager to buy one letter signed by John Hancock but everything had been organized into lots that I could not afford.

When I went to take the exams in January, I realized to my horror that I had a high fever and felt extremely unwell. I struggled through the written anatomy exam as best I could but when it came to the practical, where I had to bend over one cadaver after another, I feared I was going to faint. I staggered over to a stool and sat down with my head between my knees.

A lab instructor came over: "What's going on here?"

"I feel awful," I groaned.

She put her hand on my forehead. "You're burning up with fever. But I can't send you down to the doctor—there's a strict rule that no one can leave before the exam is over."

We were divided into small groups for the practical. The rule against leaving was to prevent the next group of students, waiting outside the lab, from benefiting from information imparted by anyone dismissed early.

The instructor stood by looking worried. "You really do look awful. Wait—I'll get someone to go with you to the infirmary. That way we'll be sure you don't talk to anyone on your way out." So much for the honor system!

The doctor, an elderly woman with a brusque manner, did a thorough exam and noted that I was jaundiced. She began prodding my liver, which was enlarged and tender. She was obviously delighted with her diagnostic acumen, because she continued prodding it again and again, as if to convince me, as I winced with pain, that the diagnosis was correct.

The viruses for hepatitis had not yet been discovered. The doctor said, "You have catarrhal jaundice. We have to flush out your liver and intestines to get rid of all the toxins."

She gave me a bottle of citrate of magnesia, which causes a profound watery diarrhea, and instructed me to drink the whole bottle. I obediently followed directions and went into shock with dehydration. I had to be hospitalized for over a week, missing the rest of the exams.

I was completely distraught and was afraid I would be flunked out. Dr. Marion Fay, dean of the medical school and our professor of biochemistry, came to the rescue. Many people feared Dr. Fay. Tall and thin to the point of gauntness, her carried herself extremely erect and seemed all-seeing and all-knowing. She was very strict and appeared humorless but I found that she was actually a very caring person. She demanded high standards but was concerned for our welfare. She visited me in the hospital and spent time reassuring me that I was a good student and had nothing to fear. She arranged for me to take make-up exams. It was difficult to show affection to a person with her degree of reserve but I felt she knew how much I liked her and that I appreciated her efforts on my behalf.

I boarded closer to the college during my second year. I lived in the home of a young couple with small children. Costs were decreased because I served as babysitter at night. The couple liked to spend their evenings at a bar and befriended an army officer who also frequented the bar. He began to spend increasing amounts of time at the house. I disliked him intensely. He walked with a swagger and boasted of his many exploits. Of medium height and somewhat rotund, he considered himself a Lothario and felt that I should be impressed with him in his officers' uniform. I went out of my way to avoid his macho attempts to further our friendship. He disappeared for several weeks, only to reappear one weekend with the announcement that he was getting married the following Sunday. Dinner that night centered on an excited discussion of the forthcoming nuptials.

The next day I was called down to the Dean's office, where two men waited to see me. They identified themselves as FBI agents and said very kindly, "Now Gloria, don't be afraid, we both have children your age and we know kids can get into trouble."

I looked at them in disbelief, not knowing what I should be afraid of or what trouble I was in. They showed me a picture of the soldier who had been coming to the house.

"Do you know this man?" they asked.

"Why, yes," I said in some surprise.

"Do you know where he is now?"

"No," I said, "I don't know where he is, but I do know where he's getting married next Sunday." They looked puzzled.

"Who is he marrying?"

"I haven't the faintest idea."

"Aren't you upset?"

"Why should I be?"

They told me he was an army private who had gone AWOL and had been picked up wearing an officer's uniform. He had escaped several days previously. While in custody, he had not mentioned the couple he had befriended but said he had been living with me. I was aghast.

"WHAT?" I exclaimed. "I had nothing to do with that man. He is absolutely NOT MY TYPE." My obvious distress must have convinced them because they became apologetic and assured me that they would notify the Dean of my innocence. They found the church where the soldier was to be married and arrested him at the altar the following week. The couple I boarded with were furious with me for being responsible for his capture. I left that house as soon as possible and moved in with Eva Reich, who had a room in a house just across the courtyard.

My friendship with Eva was closer than ever but it had its down side. She had been living for a while with a young man she had met. The school had found out about it and she was sternly reprimanded. Dr. Fay said, "We will not tolerate your cohabitation with a man unless you are married. It affects the reputation of the entire school. If you continue to flout decorum you will be expelled."

Eva had no intention of getting married and took a room by herself. She became miserable and missed her Jerry very much. It began to affect her studies and mine too when I moved in with her. After a while she decided marriage was the only solution and she and Jerry got a license to be married in a civil ceremony. Eva's father was furious and tried to prevent it but he arrived too late. Eva, Jerry and I, with several other friends, went down to City Hall in a holiday mood. They treated the whole affair as a lark. I had misgivings from the start. Jerry was a very nice, gentle young man who did social work. He was no match for Eva, who had an exceedingly overwhelming personality. It was obvious that this was a marriage of convenience. Eva moved back with Jerry and I stayed on in the room she had rented. The marriage only lasted until we graduated.

Our friendship affected our relationships at the college. Eva had always been something of a rebel and could be very tactless. Many members of the faculty disapproved of her, particularly after the episode resulting in her marriage, but she was a brilliant student and seemed oblivious of the disapproval of others. As her closest friend I was tarred with the same brush. Our pathology professor, Dr. Mollie Geiss, was a splendid teacher whom I greatly admired but she had strong likes and dislikes among the students. She disliked Eva intensely and I soon found that it extended to me even though I could think of nothing I had done to provoke her.

One day Dr. Geiss announced, "I want a research paper from each of you, due by the end of the semester. Choose a topic and schedule an appointment with me so that we can decide whether it would be suitable."

I had become interested in the work of Hans Selye, who had just published his revolutionary theory of the effects of stress on adrenal hormones and human health, and when I had my conference with Dr. Geiss I told her that was the topic I had chosen. She frowned and shook her head. "That's not for you. I've already decided to give it to another student. You can do your paper on Ayerza's Disease." Few physicians today would recognize the term. Dr. Ayerza was the pathologist who described the changes in the blood vessels of the lung that are associated with pulmonary hypertension. It was not my favorite topic. I later learned that the student chosen to write about Hans Selye's theories had never even heard of him until given that assignment.

Despite these set-backs, the second year of medical school was much better than the first. We began to have contact with patients. We learned physical diagnosis and applied our lessons in physiology to living, breathing people. Starting the clinical training was exciting and although we had no involvement in their actual care, some of us became attached to "our" patients.

One of my patients was an African-American girl, somewhat younger than I, who had far-advanced rheumatic heart disease and was in heart failure. She had been chosen for us to examine because she had a variety of heart murmurs that we had to learn to distinguish and diagnose. She was lonesome and afraid, and I would spend time trying to cheer her up. One day I found her sobbing bitterly. She had been a soloist in her church choir and had been looking forward to the following Sunday when Paul Robeson was scheduled to sing at her Baptist church. The idea of missing his concert was devastating to her. I tried to console her and suddenly had an idea. There was no way that she could still sing with the choir but perhaps I could arrange for a pass so that she could leave the hospital for a few hours to hear Robeson sing. I spoke with her private physician, Dr. James, who was quite reluctant to grant the pass. I hesitated a moment and then said tentatively, "Perhaps I could accompany her. I could check her pulse and make sure she doesn't exert herself." Dr. James looked at me for a long time as if assessing the situation. We all understood that some risk was involved but this was a very special event in Vicki's life. And none of us knew how long she could survive with her extensive heart damage, no matter how strictly she was kept at bed rest. Dr. James finally nodded. "Okay. I guess I could let her go by wheelchair. But they haven't the money for a private ambulance. They'll have to get someone with a car big enough to accommodate her." Vicki and her parents were overjoyed and found several people in the church who volunteered to transport us. They thanked me profusely. I had to admit to myself that my motives were not entirely altruistic. I was a great admirer of Paul Robeson. We had his records at home and I had seen him in movies and heard him on radio. The idea of seeing him in person was very exciting.

Vicki's parents spoke to the pastor who arranged for us to have a front pew. Vicki, her hair carefully braided, wore a pretty white dress with blue ribbons. The tumultuous beating of her heart had always been visible over her thin rib cage, but seeing her fully dressed with the heart action causing the thin dress to heave over her chest was disconcerting. My own heart began pounding. It was the first time I had taken responsibility for a patient and I suddenly felt unsure that I was ready for it.

I was the only white person in the church but didn't feel at all uncomfortable. Many people knew Vicki and knew why I was there and came forward to welcome us. I will never forget how Paul Robeson sang that day. There was a warmth between him and the congregation, a communication of love and shared feelings that couldn't be reproduced on records or any other media. The pastor had told him about Vicki and after the concert he came over to say hello and thank us for coming. He towered above us. I barely reached his shoulders, even standing in my high heels. I could feel the warmth of his handshake. His deep resonant voice was very gentle. I was quite overwhelmed by this great man.

We had another heart patient whom I will never forget. She was a very beautiful fair-haired young woman who was cheerful and did not appear very ill except for being somewhat pale. She and her private physician joked together a lot when she was introduced to us. After we had examined her and she was wheeled out of the room, he said, "That young woman will probably be dead within the month."

She had subacute bacterial endocarditis (SBE), an infection of the heart valves, for which no effective treatment existed at that time. As he explained this to us he said, "We are going to try a new medicine that has just been introduced in this country. Sir Alexander Fleming, a doctor in England, found that a certain mold of the genus Penicillium could kill bacteria. He derived a substance from the mold that he calls penicillin. I have been able to obtain a supply and we are going to give her massive doses; 5,000 units intramuscularly each day for a week."

SBE today is treated with millions of units of penicillin daily, given intravenously, usually combined with one of the newer antibiotics. The term "massive doses of 5,000 units" would be considered an oxymoron. The survival rate from SBE now is good. The "massive dose" given then was ineffectual. Our lovely young patient lived somewhat longer than the month prophesied by her doctor, but eventually began to run high fevers and died of septicemia.

Pediatrics occupied a very minor part of the curriculum during my clinical years. We had little if any contact with children. The course consisted mainly of learning the signs and symptoms of the various childhood contagious diseases and how to treat them. Since antibiotics had not as yet been discovered (except for penicillin which was not available for general use) treatment was mostly symptomatic. We did have sulfa drugs and we had to memorize a long list of the various sulfanilamide derivatives with the doses and indications for each. Since their names were very similar and their treatment indications confusing, I did not do well on examinations. I did somewhat better in remembering the schedule for immunizations since there were so few of them, just DPT (diphtheria, pertussis [whooping cough] and tetanus) and smallpox vaccination. Immunizations against measles, mumps and rubella (german measles) did not exist. There was no polio vaccine. Poliomyelitis, called infantile paralysis, occurred each summer and infected not only a large number of children, but also some adults. Our president, FDR, had been paralyzed by polio early in his political career but had continued despite profound disability.

The other part of the pediatric curriculum had to do with the vitamin deficiency diseases; how to diagnose and treat them. There were no multivitamin preparations for prevention. We learned that rickets had long been considered a contagious disease until some doctors from Harvard, vacationing at Cape Cod, heard about the fishermen's "superstition" that rickets could be prevented or cured by giving their children liver from the codfish. At first these academics laughed at such nonsense, but finally noted that the fishermen's children showed little signs of rickets in contrast to the children in Boston. They decided to test the theory and found that a substance they called vitamin D, found in the fish liver, did indeed prevent rickets. And so cod liver oil came into use. The discoveries of cures for other vitamin deficiencies were equally serendipitous. Scurvy was rife in the British navy and killed more sailors than the Napoleonic wars. A British surgeon on one of the frigates that visited Jamaica discovered that a ration of lime juice each day would prevent it. That was how British sailors came to be called "limeys." It wasn't until many years later that the active substance in citrus fruit, named vitamin C, was discovered. I was fascinated by the story of these discoveries but had difficulty and not much interest in remembering pediatric dosages for vitamins and sulfa drugs. My pediatrics professor lost patience with me. "Do me one favor," she said. "Promise me you'll never become a pediatrician!"

During my junior year, in 1946-47, expenses rose considerably. The cost of tuition was raised as well as the cost of books, room and board, and general living expenses. My parents were having increasing difficulty meeting my needs. With Dr. Fay's recommendation, I got a job as an emergency technician for both my junior and senior years, at the college hospital. I had free room and board, living on the top floor of the hospital in the intern's quarters. It was a convenient arrangement since I also had little laundry to worry about. I lived in surgical scrubs, saving my wardrobe (which consisted of my blue suit, a skirt, some blouses and a sweater) for the weekends. I did blood work and assisted with emergency procedures at night. I was on call some nights as a student and other nights as a technician, trying to study whenever I could. I was chronically sleep-deprived and learned to cat-nap during any spare moment.

All the rooms in the interns' quarters had windows opening onto a roof. At the end of the long corridor lived a former student who had been several classes ahead of me. She had experienced what was then called a "nervous breakdown" in her third year and had become violent and hallucinatory. She had been hospitalized and received electroconvulsive treatments, the only therapy known at the time. She had apparently recovered and the school had taken her back as part-time technician, part-time student. She was pleasant but reclusive. I didn't know her well.

Late one night I was returning from an emergency call when I saw her wandering down the hall barefoot, clad only in a long white nightgown. She looked like a ghost in the dim light. When she saw me she called out plaintively, "Birds! There are birds in my room! How can I sleep in a room full of birds!"

Cold chills ran down my spine. I was sure that her schizophrenia had returned and she was hallucinating. I had no idea how to deal with this but I took her by the hand and said gently, "Let's go back to your room. Maybe the birds have flown away."

As we approached the end of the corridor, I could hear the rustling of feathers and loud cooing. A flock of pigeons which had been nesting on the roof had invaded her room through the open window. We arranged for her to sleep elsewhere while her room was evacuated and thoroughly cleaned. It was my first lesson in not making snap diagnoses.

My closest friend in the interns' quarters was Carrie, a classmate who lived next door to me and had the same financial arrangement that I had. We became inseparable, sharing confidences and offering mutual support during times of stress. The only hitch in our friendship was that Carrie was a medical missionary who was determined to get me to accept Jesus. After repeated attempts without success, she broke down and began to cry. "Gloria, I can't bear the idea of you burning in hell for all eternity!"

I put my arm around her consolingly. "Carrie, please don't worry. It doesn't worry me at all."

There were many students of Carrie's persuasion, who lived strict, sheltered lives. They were very religious and did not approve of dancing, movies, or any of the other forms of entertainment that relieved the unremitting stress of our studies. They were often shocked by Eva Reich's psychoanalytic theories, which she expounded at length at lunch or social evenings at one of the "fraternities." These were women's social groups that would have been called sororities elsewhere, but that term was spurned at Women's Med. Eva liked to interpret our dreams and explain their psychosexual significance. A group would gather around her, eager to hear her evaluation of their latest dream. Carrie's group looked on with disapproval.

"My dreams have no sexual content," said one of the latter. "But I have recurring dreams related to my fear of flying. Last night, I dreamed I was in a plane that was about to crash. I had to bail out with a large white parachute. I landed on top of the Washington Monument." Eva opened her mouth to speak and I kicked her under the table. She looked at me in surprise: I was slowly shaking my head. I did not think it appropriate for her to discuss the phallic symbolism of the Washington Monument with these women. She shrugged and decided to say nothing.

Our class was divided roughly into two groups: an older, highly religious group who aspired to be medical missionaries and a younger, more worldly group that included Eva and me. Our group often lunched together or socialized at the fraternities. One day, as one of them left the lunch table, another began recounting a cruel ethnic joke relating to her Italian ancestry. I said, "Jean, please don't talk like that. It makes me wonder what you say about me, as a Jew, when I'm not around." The others looked at each other guiltily. Racial and religious bigotry was openly expressed even in polite circles.

My romantic life was extremely limited at medical school. Although I dated sporadically, none of these relationships were serious. The Cinderella complex that had developed during the years I lived with my aunt definitely affected my relationships with men. My fantasies about the ideal Prince Charming could not be equaled by any of the men I dated.

Eva Reich was quite critical and used a lot of psychiatric jargon to explain my reluctance to commit myself to a serious relationship. Although troubled by Eva's diagnosis of my psychological problems, I still stubbornly persisted in discontinuing friendships I did not enjoy. And with a full study schedule and my extra work as an emergency technician, I had little time or energy for outside romance.

Our curriculum was becoming increasingly clinical and we had night call on the various services. We assisted with deliveries on obstetrics and various emergencies throughout the hospital. In obstetrics, we graduated from delivering babies in the hospital to doing home deliveries, accompanied only by a nurse. I remember the fear of going out on my first home delivery. The nurse was much more experienced than I and walked me through it without incident. After a while I looked forward to this service with great pleasure. I never got over the wonder of bringing a new life into the world. The sense of accomplishment was overwhelming, multiplied by the family's joy and gratitude. Fortunately, I never ran into any difficulty. Home deliveries are marvelous when everything goes right. They can be a nightmare when complications arise. I do not recommend them.

With my duties as an emergency technician, I was doubly stressed. Early one morning, with little sleep the night before, I was called to assist our head of surgery with an emergency operation. Rushing to the OR without breakfast, I scrubbed, donned sterile gown and gloves, and joined the surgeon at the operating table. The procedure was a long one and I began to feel faint. I tried to fight it but felt everything going black and pitched forward. I was grabbed unceremoniously from behind. My last recollection was the surgeon roaring, "Get that woman out of here before she unsteriles my field!"

I was particularly attracted to the surgical service, and loved the instant gratification of cutting and sewing to make a patient well. While on this service, I had my first true infatuation. A young and very handsome surgeon had joined our staff and my greatest joy was to assist him at operations. One day a young couple was brought by ambulance to the Emergency Room after an auto accident. The husband was severely injured, although still conscious. The wife, only slightly bruised, was crying and holding his hand, not wanting to leave him. My handsome surgeon peremptorily ordered her out of the room. Turning to one of the nurses he said, in his flat, somewhat nasal voice,"I can't stand these emotional Jews." End of my one-sided romance.

Much of our clinical training was at Philadelphia General Hospital (PGH—a city hospital now defunct), where we shared ward service and faculty with students from the other Philadelphia medical schools—the University of Pennsylvania, Temple, Jefferson and Hahneman. It was there that I got my first taste of the contempt and harassment to which women in medicine were subject. We frequently had ward rounds with students from the other schools. The doctor leading the rounds would make derogatory remarks about the "hen medics" and how he had to simplify things for their understanding. A frequent comment was that there had never been a hen medic who knew how to dress or act attractively and any man who would consider marriage with one was not really a man. Another familiar joke was that hen medics suffered from an occupational hazard. As they pursued their careers, their ovaries atrophied.

Despite these witticisms about how unattractive we were, we had to be on guard against sexual harassment. There were many private places on the wards, corridors, and stairwells of a large hospital, and we had to be careful not to be caught alone in them. Several women in my class had unpleasant experiences but would not think of complaining. In that environment, the victim was usually the one blamed.

One particular class comes to mind, not as an example of sexual harassment as much as of the prevailing insensitivity of the time. We had a course in psychiatry held Saturday mornings in the amphitheater at PGH. It was considered great entertainment and the male students from the other schools brought their dates, beautifully dressed young women in high heels, many sporting the huge chrysanthemum corsages often worn to football games. The psychiatrist running the show demonstrated his unfortunate patients; their delusions, hallucinations, catatonic posturings, as if they were circus freaks. The general merriment was increased by his sly sexual innuendoes. One patient was a young woman who might once have been pretty but now appeared with bedraggled, dull, stringy hair and shapeless hospital gown. She had catatonic schizophrenia, with unfocussed eyes that stared into the distance. She shuffled in, led by an attendant, and did not respond to the psychiatrist's cheerful greeting or questioning.

"Catatonics can hold the same position for hours at a time," he said. He then arranged her arms and legs, like a store manikin, in a series of poses that she did not resist and which she held until he moved her again. The "audience" screamed with laughter. I did not consider this a very constructive way of teaching. I was ashamed for all of us.

During the summer between my junior and senior year I served a "clinical clerkship" at a hospital in a small town in southern Pennsylvania. Clinical clerks were medical students in their final years of training and performed the same functions as interns under closer supervision. We received a small stipend in addition to room and board and I was delighted that I had been accepted for the position.

I enjoyed the increased experience in caring for patients, and an added attraction was the presence of several other clinical clerks from Philadelphia medical schools. For the first time I felt I was treated as an equal, both by the male medical students and the supervising doctors. We worked well as a team and in the relaxed summer atmosphere we picnicked, hiked, and just enjoyed each other's company during our time off.

One member of our team was a tall, cheerful, blond young man named Tom. We soon found we shared many interests, particularly a love of music and of reading. We began to take long walks together, talking of the books we had read and our favorite composers. Tom was an excellent pianist and in the evening we would all gather in the doctor's lounge, furnished with an old beat-up piano, to hear him play. Despite its appearance, all the keys worked and it was tuned acceptably. I loved the Chopin and Mozart but most of the group could tolerate just so much of "that highbrow stuff" and so, with much laughter, we would switch to Gilbert and Sullivan and sing all the ditties with great gusto. In those days before television, every home with a piano had piles of sheet music and a favorite evening activity was singing together at the piano.

As the summer progressed, it seemed that Tom and I were becoming increasingly fond of each other. On the last weekend we went to an open air summer theater together to see The Mikado. After the show, laughing and singing some of the clever, rollicking songs ("I've Got a Little List") we strolled arm in arm to a café for coffee and dessert.

Tom suddenly became serious. "Gloria, this has been a great summer. I'm sorry it's ending." He hesitated. "And knowing you has made it really special."

I smiled and nodded. "I feel the same."

"But," he continued, "I won't be able to see you once we get back to Philadelphia."

I stiffened. "Why not?"

He blurted out, "My parents would never understand my dating a Jewish girl."

I said slowly, "I can understand your parents not wanting you to marry outside your faith. Many Jewish parents feel the same. Are you saying you can't even have Jewish friends?"

He nodded shame-facedly.

I rose from my seat slowly. I have a tendency to cry easily but was grateful that this time pride and anger kept the tears back.

"Okay. Well goodbye, then. It's been nice knowing you."

"Gloria, don't go away mad."

"I'm not mad," I lied. "Just disappointed. I thought our war against Hitler would end this sort of thing. But I guess it will go on forever."

I graduated medical school in June, 1948. Graduation was held in the Irvine Auditorium of the University of Pennsylvania, and my parents had invited the entire family—all my aunts and uncles who had so strongly disapproved of my becoming a doctor. The ceremony of conferring the MD degree is quite impressive.

We all had hooded velvet mantles, the sign of our new status, placed on our shoulders as we received our diplomas. At the end, we recited the Hippocratic Oath in unison. It was wonderful seeing my parents looking so proud and happy. We posed for a picture together, I in cap and gown holding my diploma; they, standing tall, their faces beaming. My father had arranged for all the family to have dinner together in a private room of a well-known restaurant. Taking my arm, Dad whispered, "I think this is one of the best days of my whole life." I could feel the tears filling my eyes. The struggle of the preceding four years had been justified. And we had managed it without borrowing money from the family.

As we went arm in arm to the restaurant, I noted that my father did not have the strength and vigor that I had always taken for granted. He was walking slowly, somewhat stooped, pausing frequently to catch his breath. I realized with a shock that he was getting old. He was now over sixty but had never been seen by a doctor, except to repair a deep cut made with an axe that had slipped while he was chopping wood. I said, "Dad, I think you should have a checkup. You seem to be having some trouble getting around." He laughed and shook his head. In those days one didn't see a doctor unless acutely ill.

At the end of the summer, however, he admitted that he had chest pain while walking or doing the hard manual work required at Schroon Lake. A cardiologist confirmed my worst fears. My father had severe arteriosclerotic heart disease and high blood pressure. The doctor gave him nitroglycerin tablets that relieved the chest pain and told him to "take it easy." There was little more that he could do. My father laughed ironically. "I'll have plenty of time to take it easy when I'm dead," he said. His entire livelihood depended on the hard work he did at Schroon Lake and he had no intention of stopping. I felt helpless and frustrated. I had been so proud of becoming a doctor and suddenly realized that, although my father had worked hard to put me through medical school, medicine could offer him little in return.

GLORIA O. SCHRAGER, M.D.

GRADUATION FROM MEDICAL SCHOOL

My Mother, Edith Levine Ogur and My Father, Ellis M. Ogur at My Graduation

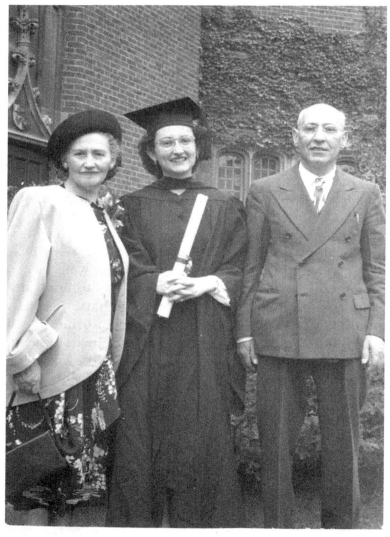

June 1948

Woman's Medical School gave me the best training available at the time but the four years were not particularly pleasant. Most of the other women, considerably older than I, had had careers in nursing or social work before deciding on medicine. The majority were unmarried and had no interest in marriage. In fact many of the faculty said marriage and a career in medicine were incompatible and anyone contemplating the two was wasting her time. Those with religious backgrounds, like Carrie, had chosen medicine so they could become medical missionaries, to go abroad and convert the heathen. They all considered me good practice material and were upset with me when I politely but firmly declined.

I decided to intern at a large hospital where I could have more experience and responsibility than at a small private hospital. I applied to many prestigious hospitals and was rejected by all of them. Very few had women on their staff. My brother Moe had collaborated on a biochemistry textbook with a professor at one of the university hospitals, and he wrote him a letter on my behalf. When I went to see the professor, he peered at me through greasy wire-rimmed glasses. He was a scrawny, nervous little man and his eyes kept shifting around the room. His hair was meticulously combed over the top of his head in a vain attempt to hide the bald spot. He kept tapping his desk with his left index finger, as if he wanted to press a button that would make me disappear. "I have never recommended a woman for a position in this hospital and I never intend to," he said. "Why should you deprive some worthy male student of a good internship?"

I was finally accepted at Metropolitan Hospital, one of New York City's municipal hospitals. It was not my first choice since it was not truly a university hospital. It was affiliated with New York Medical School but their primary teaching hospital was the Flower Fifth Avenue Hospital. However, the experience and training at Metropolitan was the equal of any. This became increasingly apparent later, when I had to sit for various Board examinations and found that I had been well prepared to perform competently.

I remember taking Part III of the National Board Examinations during my internship. The first two parts of the

National Boards were given during various stages of medical school. They were written exams testing one's knowledge, first in the basic sciences and then on the clinical curriculum. Part III was an oral examination given at a large university center. It was necessary to pass all three parts to be licensed as a physician. Part of the oral consisted of examining a patient and then discussing a differential diagnosis and how one would manage the case. I was assigned a pleasant, elderly woman who had been admitted the day before. She cooperated fully in giving me her history and allowing me to do a complete examination.

Since her complaints were principally abdominal and since the importance of a rectal examination had always been emphasized, I did one and could feel a hard, annular constricting mass at the tip of my finger. I felt surprised that they had given me such a straightforward case but became increasingly nervous when I went to the conference room and met the professor, cloaked in his starched, pure white coat emblazoned with the university insignia, waiting to discuss the case with me.

I was the only woman taking the exam that day and he gave an audible sigh when he saw me. It was unnerving. I related the history of my patient's complaints in a faltering voice and then paused. "Yes" he said impatiently, "and then what would you do?"

I blurted out, "I'd get a surgical consult." I assumed that he knew the woman's diagnosis and due to my general unease I had skipped a few steps ahead, forgetting that proper procedure required me to describe the results of my physical examination. He looked at me as if I were an idiot.

He said sarcastically, "Wouldn't you want to do something else first? A physical examination? Some tests?"

"Of course I would do a physical, and then I would call the surgeon," I answered.

"What about a differential diagnosis? Ordering some tests?" he prompted.

"But I know the diagnosis. She has an annular constricting carcinoma of the rectum," I murmured.

"And how do you know that?"

"Because I could feel it when I did my rectal exam. Before we order tests, I think we should discuss it with the surgeon."

He looked at me strangely and then began flipping through the patient's medical chart, noting the history, physical, and the long list of orders written by the admitting resident. Obviously, a rectal examination had not been done.

Without a word he picked up a rubber glove and went to the woman's bedside with me trailing meekly behind. He gently told her that part of the exam had to be repeated. When he was finished he stripped off the glove, walked out of the room, and said to me, "You are quite right, doctor. The woman does have a rectal carcinoma." He turned to one of the nurses. "Would you please page Dr. X (the admitting resident) and tell him I want to speak with him immediately." I passed the exam.

CHAPTER SIX

Metropolitan Hospital

M etropolitan Hospital, one of New York City's largest, was situated on Welfare Island (now called Roosevelt Island) in the middle of the East River. The island is long and narrow and stretches roughly from the 50's to the 80's in Manhattan. Only ambulances were permitted; private cars were forbidden on the island. Pedestrians had to use a ferry, a little tugboat contraption that slid sideways across the currents from its dock at the foot of 76th street. The aerial tramway that exists today had not yet been built.

The city had several institutions on the island. City Hospital was situated on the southern end and Metropolitan Hospital was on the northern end. Both were acute care hospitals that alternated the days that they admitted patients. Both were terribly overcrowded. In the middle of the island, close to the 57th Street (Queensboro) bridge, was Goldwater Memorial Hospital, a chronic disease hospital. The "Girls' Camp", a euphemism for a detention center for delinquent young women, was situated between Goldwater and Metropolitan. Many had sexually transmitted diseases as well as malnutrition, tuberculosis, and a host of other problems. The interns at either City Hospital or Metropolitan were responsible for treating them when they became acutely ill.

Early in the morning of the last day in June, 1948, I took the island ferry to Metropolitan to start my internship. The boat was filled with young people making one of the most difficult transitions in their lives, from students to physicians with responsibility for their patients' welfare. Many knew each other from school and were lending moral support with all kinds of off-color witticisms. I sat alone, my attention suddenly focused on a very tall, lean young man who lounged casually against one of the bulkheads. He was carrying a large thin package, like a big picture frame, carefully wrapped in brown paper. I couldn't decide whether he was a new intern or just making a delivery. He had a confident air of good humor and intelligence that made me feel instinctively he was more likely to be an intern than a delivery boy. He fit my concept of a typical Texan, or at least the movie version of one. He reminded me of Gary Cooper.

When the ferry docked on the island, we newcomers discovered that Metropolitan consisted of several buildings situated in different areas of the large campus. We walked up from the dock to a point where the path split in several directions. There were signs with arrows indicating where each path led, but none was relevant to interns' registration. Everyone hesitated, trying to decide the path to take. A self-appointed leader said confidently, "I'm sure it's this way."

All obediently trouped after him but I paused. I wanted to make up my own mind. The "Texan" came up behind me and said, "Let's not follow the crowd." I nodded, and we walked down a different path. As I had suspected, he was a new intern like the rest of us, an observant Jew from Newark who had gone to medical school in Texas through a quirk of fate engineered by the army. The large package he carried was his framed diploma from the University of Texas School of Medicine, in Galveston. We were all required to bring our original diplomas when we registered, and of course Texas had the biggest of the lot.

This was the first of many walks we would take together. For this was Alvin Schrager, whom I was to marry several years later after a stormy courtship. Al towered above me (he was over 6'4"), and walked with the easy grace of a natural athlete. He had humorous gray-green eyes and a thick mop of unruly, sandy hair that seemed in constant need of combing. He wore his clothes carelessly but still maintained an air of elegance. His wry, self-deprecating sense of humor was in stark contrast to the macho airs of many of the other interns. I was attracted to him instantly and was pleased that he asked me to join him for lunch at the staff house. This became a habit. He frequently waited for me so that we could eat together.

The dining room at the staff house was a large, airy room with many windows and round tables that seated about ten people. It was not a cafeteria. We were waited on by a cheerful staff who always checked to see that the white linen tablecloths and napkins were fresh. The staff house was a pleasant building that reminded me of an old-fashioned hotel. It had a huge front porch, many rocking chairs, and was surrounded by a beautiful lawn that stretched down to the river. We all ate there but only the male doctors lived there. The women were housed in the spare brick nurses' quarters several blocks away.

As the days went on, one of the other interns, a stocky, well-muscled young man, wanted to prove to me that my interest in Al was ill-advised.

"These tall guys are usually a push-over" he said. "I'm a lot shorter, but I bet I could throw him easily. I was on the wrestling team at college."

He challenged Al to a wrestling match on the front lawn of the staff house. He didn't know that Al had wrestled with his older brother since childhood and had also been part of a wrestling team during his army training. With a quick feint, Al had him on his back before he knew what had happened. He got up, bellowing like a bull, and charged again. Al neatly sidestepped and threw him a second time. No one challenged him after that.

As our relationship grew, Al told me that he expected the woman he married to give up her job and take care of home and children, as was the custom of the time. I told him that under no circumstances would I leave my career in medicine. He couldn't understand why I was so stubborn. His older brother, Harold, had married a graduate of Columbia Law School who had happily quit her practice to become a full-time housewife. After many fruitless discussions, we decided there was no future in our relationship and stopped going out together.

I began to date other men. One of them was a resident in Internal Medicine at Bellevue Hospital, who was distantly related to my family. The chief of his service invited the resident staff, with their spouses or "a friend" to his house for a dinner each year, and Burt asked me to go with him. His chief was married to a prominent TV personality and lived in a penthouse on Sutton Place, reached by private elevator. I was excited at the thought of dining in such elegant surroundings, and splurged most of my miniscule savings on a new dress. Christian Dior had just introduced The New Look—a fashion which emphasized a tiny waist and flared out to a full skirt of ballerina length. It was a reaction to the clothes rationing of the war. Since I had a small waist, it was a style that fit me well and I was ready to sacrifice a great deal to wear such a dress.

Sutton Place, bordering the East River, is one of the most prestigious residential areas in Manhattan. I wore the Christian Dior copy with a pearl necklace and earrings and felt very elegant as the doorman ushered us into the imposing lobby. My self-confidence suddenly disappeared when I met my host and hostess. I was overawed by the sophisticated company. I was afraid of appearing gauche through some inappropriate remark and became tongue-tied and miserable. My shyness went completely unnoticed. The TV star dominated the conversation and all we had to do was smile and nod. When it came time to sit down for dinner, she trilled: "I have a wonderful treat for you. I have just stolen the chef from my best friend and he makes simply mahhhvelous exotic Near-Eastern dishes."

She signaled and the chef proudly brought in a large, covered silver platter. As he removed the cover with a flourish, a familiar odor assailed my nostrils. "This," said our hostess, "is called Kay-Shah." It was kasha varnichkas, a very common Jewish dish that my mother frequently prepared for the family. It was one of the very few foods that I detested.

I did not flaunt my social activities but I did not hide them either. Al heard about them and he was furious. After a while we had an emotional reconciliation. This silly pattern of behavior was repeated many times, each episode ending in a heated argument, with Al stalking off and me in tears. But that day in June when we first met, all was sunny and serene, and it was the start of a beautiful if rocky friendship.

There were just two or three women among the intern and resident staff in a house staff that numbered close to a hundred if one counted all the residents and fellows. The idea of the staff house being co-ed was unthinkable, and the women were exiled to the nurse's quarters a couple of blocks from the main hospital. Unlike the men, we had no phones in our rooms. Pagers were still science fiction in a Dick Tracy comic strip. There was just one phone in the hall. When its clamor woke us at night, we'd pull the covers over our heads and wait with bated breath while the night watchman came slowly clumping down the hall on his artificial leg to knock loudly on the door of the luckless intern called for an emergency. Each night had these multiple interruptions but I can't say they seriously interfered with my slumber. As soon as I knew the call wasn't for me, I'd sigh with relief and drop back to unconsciousness in an instant. When you're chronically sleep-deprived, your body learns to take advantage of every precious moment.

RuthEllen Steinman was the only other woman among the new group of interns. She had the room next to mine and we became close friends. We all called her Ruthie. She came from a family of physicians. Her mother was a GP and her older brother, Bob Steinman, was a resident in internal medicine, several years ahead of us. Ruthie had a totally irreverent sense of humor and was an accomplished mimic. I was still in great awe of the attending staff, some of whom were quite pompous. Ruthie soon cured me of that. The way she could imitate their idiosynchrasies was quite devastating and she often had me doubled up with laughter.

Ruthie had a seemingly inexhaustible store of energy. She was short and stocky and never walked—she always ran. She could swear as volubly as any of the men. We shared our worries and troubles, and her cheerful way of dispatching with them all by a couple of well-chosen epithets made the stresses of internship easier to bear.

Metropolitan Hospital was one of New York City's oldest, its wards crowded with the poorest of the poor. It had a certain Dickensian quality about it. In fact Charles Dickens, visiting America in the 1840's, had seen it and had written about the dreadful conditions—and little had changed since. But he had described the broad, graceful spiral staircase that wound up the three flights of the huge central hall in the main building. One had to admire its beauty despite the sordid surroundings.

The wards all led off this main area, so crowded that beds were in the halls and every other available space. The admitting area was in the dank basement, with exposed, leaking pipes above the patients' beds. New patients couldn't be sent to the wards until someone died or was discharged (the probabilities were about equal). Interns have often complained, rightfully so, about the conditions under which they worked but I believe that Metropolitan Hospital was in a class by itself.

The main building housed the medical and surgical adult patients. There were separate buildings for pediatrics and obstetrics, for the laboratories and for tuberculosis (TB) patients. As a rotating intern, my training was in all these areas. Few training programs today offer that kind of first year program. Medical students have to pick their field of specialization before they graduate. I think this is unfortunate. The extra year's experience in a variety of fields makes one more sure of one's interests.

I enjoyed all the services but my favorite was surgery. I loved the drama of the operating room and my last two years of medical school, assisting as an emergency technician, made me more experienced in the OR than most of the other interns. The surgeons appreciated this and I was offered a much-coveted residency in surgery. I was delighted and flattered. A young surgeon who had become a good friend took me aside and said, "Think twice before you accept. Sure, the attending surgeons like you to assist them. But which one of them will offer to take a woman as a partner in his private practice after she graduates from the program? And what chance would you have setting up a surgical practice on your own?"

I remembered the few women surgeons I had known at Women's Medical College, a place mostly free of sexual bias. I didn't envy their life styles. They seemed to have few interests aside from their work, except for Dr. Alma Dea Morani, who was an accomplished sculptor. None of them appeared to be married or have any family life. With great reluctance and hesitation, I finally declined the offer.

I was also fond of the pediatrics service. In medical school, although we had learned the rudiments of this specialty, our actual contact with young patients had been very limited. I found now that working with children was a great pleasure. I had the same feeling of instant gratification that had attracted me to surgery but it was of a different nature. You might admit a desperately ill child one day, start the appropriate treatment, and return the next day to find the child laughing and jumping around in the crib. As one of the pediatricians put it, "Mother Nature is on your side when you treat kids."

One of the most hazardous services was on the TB pavilion. Antibiotics for TB, such as streptomycin, had just been discovered and their use was limited. The building was crowded to capacity with patients who had advanced disease. The main treatment consisted of pneumothorax, a procedure in which air is inserted into the chest cavity with a needle to collapse the lung so it would "rest." If that didn't work several ribs would be cut away to expose the lung and the diseased part would be surgically removed. Interns performed the pneumothorax procedure almost daily. We were supervised the first few times but then we were on our own. We also assisted at all surgery and were responsible for the post-operative care. We would have to irrigate (wash out) the open, draining wounds. The lung was clearly visible when we washed away the quantities of caseous, purulent material swarming with live tubercle bacilli.

We fluoroscoped patients daily in a small, windowless, poorly ventilated room. It was no bigger than a walk-in closet, accommodating about six people at the most. This included the several patients to be examined. The rule about wearing face masks was only casually observed by both patients and doctors.

Fluoroscopy is similar to X-ray except that you do not get a permanent image on film. You see the image on a screen, in real time. It is possible to see the heart beating and how the lung functions with each breath. The screen emits much radiation. With present technology, the radiologist isn't in the room when that kind of imaging is done. There is a monitor outside, and the room is constructed to prevent the escape of radiation. Back then, the dangers of radiation were largely unknown and a group of us would gather in the small fluoroscopy room without any protection.

The senior resident demonstrated the extent of disease in the patients waiting to be fluoroscoped. He kept his foot on the pedal of the fluoroscope for long periods of time so that the screen would remain lit while we checked the progress in each patient. We learned a lot about anatomy and TB this way but were ignorant of the radiation damage that might be happening to our own bodies. In addition to this hazard, the constant exposure to active tuberculosis caused most of us to develop positive TB skin tests. Our own immune systems had to fight the disease. TB prophylaxis did not exist. Some of the interns came down with the active disease.

I also had to ride the ambulance. The year before, a medical technician had made the inexcusable error of pronouncing an ambulance patient dead, only to have him sit up later in the morgue. The scandal made huge headlines and the Mayor decreed that doctors had to go on all ambulance calls. The area covered by Metropolitan stretched from the posh residences on Sutton Place to Harlem tenements. Regulations stated that the ambulance driver and the police were to accompany doctors to all emergencies. I noted they were always prompt to assist on calls to the Sutton Place area but somewhat slower to make their appearance in Harlem. I often climbed dimly lit, rat-infested, rotting staircases alone, dragging the heavy emergency medical bag without help. I don't remember any feeling of fear. My white uniform created a sense of invulnerability. And in truth, nothing frightening ever happened. Some of my most pleasant memories were delivering babies under primitive conditions in these tenements with a happy, grateful family gathered around, pressing me to eat their homemade delicacies.

The ambulance reached the island by an elevator located in one of the pylons of the Queensboro (57th Street) Bridge. The elevator was enclosed in a building at bridge level. The building also had a garage for the ambulances, an on-call dormitory for the interns, and an office with a desk and phone where the ambulance drivers kept a log book of calls. A pot of very strong, very hot coffee sat on one side of the desk and was constantly replenished. It was in great demand to help us get through the long, hectic nights. The interns' dormitory was a small windowless room with several cots placed close together. When we came back from a call, we would throw ourselves indiscriminately on whatever cot was empty. It was the one area of the hospital where sleeping accommodations were co-ed, but the hospital authorities did not seem concerned. If they thought about it at all they probably realized that we were all so exhausted, the only thing on our minds was to get as much sleep as possible between calls.

Although sleep-deprived, I remember the excitement and delight of making ambulance calls as the sun rose and the ambulance descended from the heights of the bridge. The city looked so beautiful and clean and golden in the dawn. Wide-awake despite little sleep, I wished I was an artist or a poet to capture the beauty of the sight.

One day I went on an ambulance call to a Manhattan police station. They had just captured an escaped prisoner who had killed a policeman. His scalp was bleeding profusely from a deep wound he had sustained in the struggle leading to his arrest. After I disinfected the area and controlled the bleeding, I filled a syringe with a local anesthetic and prepared to inject it before stitching. One of the policeman growled, "Don't bother with the anesthetic, doc, he's just an animal."

I replied quietly, "I'm sure he'll get the punishment he deserves. But I always use an anesthetic before sewing up any human being." When I finished, I gently cleansed the blood from his head and his face. During all this time the prisoner, a giant of a man, had sat stoically silent, head bent, manacled to a chair. As I cleaned the blood from his face our eyes met for the first time. We were both expressionless, and yet—

It was on one of these ambulance calls that I learned that cause and effect were not as straightforward as they sometimes seemed. I was called to see a woman who was having a severe asthmatic attack. She was elderly and obese and was having great difficulty breathing. Emergency treatment for severe asthma at that time consisted in giving intravenous aminophylline. It could be very effective but it also could be dangerous. One had to calculate the dose carefully and inject it very slowly. I had just cleansed her arm in preparation for inserting the needle into her vein when the woman gasped and stopped breathing. Our attempts to resuscitate her were unsuccessful. If this had occurred a moment later when the needle was in her vein, I would have been convinced that I had caused her death.

In general, internship was a constant state of fatigue. But I found this time exciting, marking not only my development as a doctor but my growth as an adult. At first the idea of having responsibility for another person's health and well-being was quite daunting. After a while you accept the fact that patients have faith in your ability and it increases your self-confidence. I was still a young woman in my twenties with all the usual insecurities, but I learned to control these emotions and project an air of reassurance for the sake of my patients. I still believe that a doctor's confidence and sympathy are powerful medicine. The constant daily crises certainly did transform us quickly from inexperienced house staff to sophisticated young doctors who had "seen this, done that." This was probably more likely in a large charity hospital than it would have been if I had interned in a small private hospital.

At the end of my internship, after I turned down the offer of a surgical residency, I accepted a residency in pediatrics and stayed at Metropolitan for three more years. Many of my friends left to continue their medical careers elsewhere. Ruthie Steinman had met a young man who was a Rhodes Scholar, just returned from England. His name was Ed Bloustein and he was about to start law school. He and Ruthie married after a relatively short courtship and Ruthie stopped her postgraduate training to open a general practice which helped support them while Ed was in law school. We lost track of one another until many years later, when Ruthie called with astounding news: Ed Bloustein had just been appointed president of Rutgers University and they were moving to New Jersey! We had a wonderful reunion and remained friends for many years. They are both gone now and I miss them.

Al had accepted a fellowship in cardiology with Dr. William Dock, a feisty, plain-spoken leader in cardiac research, at the Downstate Medical Center in Brooklyn. We saw one another much less frequently, but still occasionally called in the evenings.

We were both fatigued and overworked, and long evening phone calls were a luxury neither of us could afford.

My start as a pediatric resident was inauspicious. All the other pediatric residents were men and I did not become close friends with any of them. They assumed my relationship with Al had ended and they were less than sympathetic. Our senior resident was a tall arrogant man who openly boasted of his search for a rich wife whose parents would set him up in a Park Avenue practice. His search was successful and a lavish wedding was planned, to be held at the Waldorf-Astoria. Several weeks before the wedding, he announced that he had called it off. The pre-nuptial agreement had included an expensive new car. He had specified the precise style and make and he was furious because they had presented him with a less expensive model. They hurriedly rectified their egregious error and the happy couple proceeded to the altar on schedule.

Although I had little social contact with the other residents, we worked together well. Many of our patients were recent immigrants from the Caribbean and suffered from a host of tropical diseases with which I was unfamiliar. One morning while making rounds I noted a long tube-like structure, like the tourniquets we used to draw blood, in one of the of cribs where a child was sleeping peacefully. "Someone has been negligent," I thought. "Leaving a tourniquet lying in a child's crib is potentially dangerous." I picked it up and it began to squirm wildly in my hand. It was an ascaris, a large worm that commonly infects children in tropical climates.

The role of pediatricians in general hospitals was much more limited than it is now. Many children's diseases, such as heart or kidney problems or diabetes were treated by specialists trained to care for these diseases in adults. Training programs in pediatric subspecialties were just beginning to be organized in large university hospitals. Although pediatricians were usually responsible for the care of premature infants, obstetrician looked after the full-term babies they delivered.

I was leaving the premature nursery one day when I saw some doctors gathered around the crib of a full-term baby in the normal newborn nursery. I entered and peered on tip-toe over the shoulders of the group of men discussing the case. Obstetricians seemed particularly intolerant of woman physicians and I had the sense that I was unwelcome. My view of the baby was partially obstructed by the hulking forms who ignored my presence. The baby was jaundiced, and I learned that the tests for blood incompatibilities, which are the most frequent cause of jaundice in the newborn, had been normal. The doctors had reached the conclusion that the baby had a liver problem, probably an obstruction of the bile ducts, and they were preparing to operate.

From the limited view I had behind them all, the front of the baby's head looked swollen. I ventured timidly, "I think he has a bulging fontanelle. He may have meningitis." (The fontanelle is the "soft spot" just above a baby's forehead. It bulges when an infant has meningitis, which causes increased pressure in the brain.) The obstetricians had been so busy examining his liver that no one had paid attention to his head. They looked at me with open hostility, but one of them muttered, "We'd better do a spinal tap." Normally, spinal fluid is as clear as water. This tap was cloudy. The baby was infected with a type of bacteria, *Escherichia coli*, that causes significant jaundice in newborns. The operation on the liver was cancelled.

We had six wards located on the three floors of the pediatrics pavilion, two wards to a floor. The main floor was devoted to an admitting unit and an intensive care unit. The wards on the upper floors were devoted to the treatment of children who had diseases rarely seen today. One entire ward was crowded with children who had either acute rheumatic fever or rheumatic heart disease. There was little we could do to prevent or treat either. Penicillin was still not generally available to treat streptococcal throat infections and its role in preventing rheumatic fever, which developed in a small fraction of untreated strep throats, was unknown. If patients developed the exquisitely painful arthritis of rheumatic fever, we gave them aspirin. It was very effective in relieving the pain and swelling, but did nothing to prevent damage to the heart. The only treatment for the heart disease was digitalis, given if the heart valves were so damaged that the child went into heart failure.

Another ward was occupied by children with tuberculosis. Although it occurred among the malnourished, poverty-stricken children in this country, it was more common among recent immigrants. Most of the children recovered without any treatment except good food. There were no antibiotics that were effective against TB, except streptomycin, only available for the critically ill. I remember a little girl, Sophia, who went home apparently cured. She caught measles from her older brother and came back critically ill. Apparently the measles virus depresses a child's general immunity to TB. It also causes an inflammation of the lungs which reactivates the infection. Sophia developed miliary tuberculosis (the spread of the disease throughout her body) and died of TB meningitis.

Dr. Kurt Lange, a kidney specialist, was conducting research on kidney diseases in children and asked me to assist him. I had to spend extra hours doing tests in the lab, collecting blood, and keeping records on the patients we were treating. But it was fascinating work and I enjoyed doing it. Lange was studying the effects of cortisone on various kidney conditions. We noted that some cases of nephrotic syndrome responded dramatically to treatment while others did not. In this syndrome, the kidney cannot retain the body's protein and it is lost in the urine. The level of protein in the blood falls and water moves from the blood into the body's tissues, causing swelling (edema). Sometimes so much water accumulated in a child's belly that it became grossly swollen and we had to insert a needle to drain it. We could not understand why some of the children seemed to be cured after treatment with cortisone while others did not respond at all. One of the non-responders was a little boy named Frankie whose face and body were grotesquely swollen, to the great distress of us all.

One Sunday, I was standing at the nurse's station on the kidney ward when I noted that the curtains were pulled around Frankie's bed.

I asked the nurse in alarm, "Has anything happened to Frankie?"

She shook her head. "His parents and an uncle are visiting him. I guess they must have pulled the curtains."

As I approached the bed, I heard low singing and clicking sounds, like those made by castanets. Pulling aside the curtains, I saw Frankie staring wide-eyed at his "uncle," who had donned a headdress and necklace of brightly colored feathers. He was shaking some bones over Frankie and chanting unintelligibly.

They all looked up, startled, when they saw me. I smiled, waved my hand, said "Carry on," and closed the curtains. Grinning, I went back to the nurse and said, "Do you know what's going on back there? A witch doctor is trying to cure Frankie."

The nurse picked up the phone. "I'm going to call Security."

"No, don't do that," I said. "We haven't had much luck treating him. Let's give the witch doctor a chance."

The next day Frankie started to diurese (lose the accumulated fluid that had made him swollen) and soon looked like a normal little boy. Lange was delighted with his recovery. We were reporting our results in several medical journals, and Frankie was listed with the patients who had responded to cortisone. "I don't know," I said doubtfully. "I don't think we're giving enough credit to the witch doctor."

During these years, (1948-1951) more attention was focused on saving premature infants, and new technology was introduced. At Metropolitan we were still using a primitive incubator. It was little more than a square box with a thermostat for controlling temperature, a tube to admit oxygen and a lid on top. I learned that Babies Hospital at Columbia had just acquired the latest equipment and I requested an elective rotation to go there and learn the features of their new type of incubator. It was very impressive. It had the ability to raise the oxygen concentration in the incubator to 100%, which was thought to be of great help to premature infants who were having trouble breathing.

When I returned to Metropolitan, I tried to raise the concentrations in our incubators to 100% by sealing the lids with tape, which could be easily undone when we wanted to tend to the baby. Try as I might, leakage always occurred around the seal and it was impossible to get the oxygen concentration over 40%. I felt very frustrated and inadequate because we could not deliver the same level of care as Babies' Hospital. I felt even more frustrated because they were regularly diagnosing an eye disease of premature infants, called retrolental fibroplasia (RLF), and we were not able to diagnose a single case. This condition involved the retina and I assumed that our instruments for viewing the retina were inadequate. The retina, which lines the back of the eyeball, is like the film of a camera. Nerves record the image and transport it to the brain. If the retina is damaged, blindness can result. The cause of RLF (now called retinopathy of prematurity, ROP) was unknown at that time. Many thought it was the inevitable result of prematurity. Others thought it was a side effect of some medication we had used. It wasn't until years later that the toxic effect of high concentrations of oxygen was discovered. I had all the evidence right in front of me, but didn't have the insight to realize its significance. When the toxic effects of oxygen were recognized, the amount of oxygen given these babies was cut back severely. This caused anoxia, inadequate oxygen, which resulted in brain damage. Like so many other things in medicine, too much of a good thing could be bad but too little could be even worse.

ROP is still with us today because there are many factors other than oxygen levels that can cause the disease. But the number of cases has been reduced dramatically. Unfortunately, lawyers jumped at the opportunity to sue doctors on behalf of babies who had been damaged by too little or too much oxygen. This damage had occurred before doctors had the knowledge about how oxygen should be regulated. But when a damaged child is brought into a court room, a jury often feels that someone must pay. Many lawyers made huge fortunes in litigation over these cases. The fact that the doctors involved had worked unceasingly to save the lives of these babies, born very prematurely, was often not considered.

When I was in training, child abuse did not receive much attention. During my final year of residency the ambulance brought in two children in the last stages of starvation. They had been chained by their mother in a back room of their apartment. This was her revenge against their father, who she discovered having an affair with another woman. The couple had four children. The two who were named for the mother's family were properly fed and clothed. She had vented her rage on the two who were named for the father's family. The little boy died within hours of being admitted. The little girl was responding slowly to intravenous treatment. The Scielzo case made sensational headlines in all the New York newspapers. It was one of the first cases of child abuse reported in our area. Several days after the children were admitted, the father, a huge, burly man, appeared with some very muscular friends. "I'm signing out my kid," he said. "Where is she?"

"You can't take her," I said. "She is still too sick."

He became very threatening. I picked up the phone and asked to speak to the medical director. He wasn't available but I got through to the assistant director and told him the problem. "Is she still on the critical list?" he asked. I had to admit that she was recovering nicely and was no longer considered critical. "Then we have no right to keep the child," he said. "You'd better let her go."

I hung up the phone, looked straight at the group of threatening men, and lied. "The medical director is sending over a squad of police and security officers to arrest you. You'd better get out of here while you can."

One of the muscular friends said, "Look, we don't want no trouble", and urged the father to leave.

The next day the medical director called me. He was greatly agitated and roared over the phone, "We've just received a court order to keep that girl. If you let the father take her, you're in big trouble." I calmly reassured him that she was still with us.

I finished my pediatrics residency at Metropolitan, in June, 1951, and, since I had published research with Dr. Lange, I was offered a fellowship at New York Hospital—Cornell Medical College with Dr. Henry Barnett, who was also investigating the nephrotic syndrome. I accepted, although the amount I would be making, $100/month, did not include room and board. It was in effect a cut in pay. But I moved in with my parents in their Brooklyn apartment, so I had a little more pocket money.

My mother, who had so opposed the idea of her daughter becoming a doctor, was now reconciled and proud. She and my father had met Al and were delighted with him. Their only concern was our frequent breakups. I tried to keep my rocky romance private but they could always tell when I became silent and miserable.

One day, they approached me hesitantly. They were greatly troubled by a conversation they had just had with my aunt. She had said with great certainty that Al would never marry me. Young doctors were looking for wives from wealthy families who could supply a large dowry to set them up in practice. My father said, "Find out how much of a dowry Al wants. We'll get the money somehow."

Memories of the pediatric senior resident and his search for a rich wife came rushing back and I was furious. "So my aunt thinks you have to buy me a husband! Well, tell her that if Al was interested in a dowry I wouldn't be interested in him. Look, I can't promise you that Al and I will ever resolve our problems but I can assure you that the problem of a dowry isn't one of them." My aunt had not considered the fact that, as a physician, I would be bringing to a marriage as much financial value as my husband.

CHAPTER SEVEN

Cornell, The Red Cross, the Korean War, McCarthyism

I was 27 years old when I started my fellowship at Cornell, in 1951. Most of the women of my age were married and had children and my mother's fears about having a spinster daughter were returning. I still saw Al, although his fellowship at Downstate Medical Center in Brooklyn and my fellowship at Cornell in Manhattan gave us little time together.

Dr. William Dock, his director, was engaged in an intensive cardiac research project and kept his fellows working long hours, even on weekends. He was a brilliant, energetic, temperamental man who could be abrasive with both colleagues and students. But he had a special affection for his fellows. Although he was very demanding, he was always there, working with them. Dr. Dock was one of the first to point out the relationship between cholesterol and heart disease. A low-cholesterol diet was an obsession with him. He kept an eagle eye on what his fellows ate when they lunched together and lectured Al about his steady diet of hard-boiled eggs. (Al kept strictly kosher and there was little else in the hospital cafeteria that he could eat.) Al soon observed that Dr. Dock usually had ice cream for dessert. One day he summoned up his courage:

"Dr. Dock, I believe ice cream has more cholesterol than eggs. But you eat it every day. Can you explain your reason?"

Dock glared at him and snapped, "Why? Because I like ice cream, that's why!" His eyes sparkled and he grinned guiltily like a schoolboy caught with his hand in the cookie jar.

The Korean war had begun and legislation was passed to draft unmarried male doctors who were not in an essential position. A fellowship which involved postgraduate training in research was not considered essential and Al received his orders that October, although he had already seen service in WW II.

Shortly before he had to report to the army, he called to say he had gotten tickets for a Broadway show. "We're going to see Carol Channing in *Gentlemen Prefer Blondes*" he said. "You know how I like that song, "Diamonds are a Girl's Best Friend". I was too dense to take the hint. At dinner before the show, he took a little jewel box from his pocket and slipped the ring on my finger. It was a simple Tiffany-cut diamond and very beautiful. "I hope it fits" he said. "I decided that your ring finger was just a bit smaller than my pinky." It fit perfectly.

We knew it would be too late to avoid the draft by marrying since Al already had his orders. Besides, he was basically against the idea of a quick marriage followed by a long separation. He was going into an area of danger and he felt that marriage should wait until he returned. He was still concerned about how my medical career would interfere with family life and children. "Look, the important thing is that we love each other and can't think of a life without one another. We'll work things out somehow when I get back," he said.

One of the most bittersweet memories of my life was the New Year's Eve before Al's departure for Korea. Knowing my love of opera, he had spent a fortune on tickets to Die Fledermaus at the old Met on 38th street. This was the first time the Met had offered Fledermaus as a New Year's Eve program, the start of a long tradition. After the finale we drank champagne and joined the company in singing Auld Lang Syne. We walked in the falling snow to a turbulent Times Square at 42nd Street to see the ball come down, bringing in the New Year. Al kept his arm around me, protecting me from the surging, celebrating crowds. Two days later he flew overseas.

My fellowship at Cornell involved intensive research on the nephrotic syndrome. It was fascinating work but paid very little. Dr. Barnett suggested that I apply for a government research grant and was very pleased when it was approved. But it was not funded. This was the government's way of giving you a pat on the head for thinking up a good idea, which might further your academic career. But they did not give you the money to carry it out. It was true that research funds were sharply curtailed during the Korean War and many research projects lost their funding.

With prospects of marriage in the near future, it was necessary to look for something that would pay more than the coolie wages hospitals gave to young doctors. I knew that neither Al's parents nor mine could help us financially. In fact, there was the strong probability that they would become dependent on us for financial support before too long. My father who had been such a strong and independent man was now severely debilitated by heart disease and my mother was having a difficult time nursing him at home. Al's father had heart and lung problems. Both he and his wife were heavy smokers and it was taking its toll.

When my grant was not funded, I told Dr. Barnett that I could not continue with that level of income. He understood and wished me well. Another young doctor took over my research project. He eventually became a famous pediatric nephrologist.

I took a better-paying job with the American Red Cross Blood Center in Manhattan, going out with units to supervise blood donations. After a time, they asked me to become medical director of the Red Cross blood center in downtown Brooklyn. The center was not only responsible for donations from the borough but also collected blood on board the ships in port at the Brooklyn Navy Yard. The Yard was a hive of activity during the Korean war and its personnel were more than generous in organizing blood drives.

One day we were setting up a unit on an aircraft carrier when a sailor approached and said, "Begging your pardon ma'am, the captain's compliments and would you join him in the officer's mess." I followed dutifully, heart pounding, and was confronted by two very large, very angry men. One was the captain of the ship, the other the commander of the flight unit stationed on board. The captain was adamant that regulations prohibited pilots from flying for twenty-four hours after they had given blood. The commander said he would brook no interference with his schedule and his men were going to keep to their regular training routine. They both glared at me, expecting me to settle the dispute.

Still in my twenties, dwarfed by these two imposing, uniformed hulks, I felt totally intimidated but knew I couldn't show it. After a moment's thought, I turned to the flight commander and smiled sweetly. "I agree with you, Commander, that your pilots are men who are strong enough to fly after giving a pint of blood. However, accidents do happen and if anything untoward were to occur we would be in violation of regulations and held accountable." He grunted, shrugged his shoulders, and stalked out of the cabin. Breathing a sigh of relief, I returned to the unit

Newspapers had published articles about my appointment as medical director of the Brooklyn branch of the Red Cross late in 1952. My education and background had been mentioned and Dr. Harry Gideonse, President of Brooklyn College, was delighted by the favorable publicity for the college. He posted the clipping on his bulletin board.

This was the era of the McCarthy Committee for Un-American Activities. My brother Moe had been active in the Teachers' Union. His best friend, who was also active in organizing teachers to join the union, was called before the committee and broke down under questioning. He was handed a list of union members and asked if they were all communists. Scarcely looking at it, he nodded "yes." Moe's name was on the list. Gideonse called Moe to his office and told him he had two options. He could testify, naming more names, or he could refuse, invoking the Fifth Amendment. If he chose the latter he would be fired, even though he had tenure. Gideonse added, "It would probably involve your sister as well. It would destroy her career with the Red Cross. After all, the Navy Yard is an area of high security."

Moe, deeply troubled, spoke to me. "I'm going to refuse to testify. I'm sorry that this might affect you."

I tried to reassure him. "Do what you think is right. This whole McCarthy witch-hunt is ridiculous and one of the stupidest things about it is guilt by association. I've been totally apolitical; I've never had the time to be anything else. If the Red Cross decides to fire me, which I doubt, I could always get a job elsewhere." My picture quickly disappeared from the President's bulletin board.

The Picture Dr. Harry Gideonse, President of Brooklyn College, Hastily Removed from His Bulletin Board During the McCarthy Hearings 1951

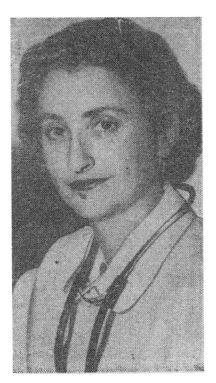

APPOINTED — Dr. Gloria Ogur, Brooklyn-born physician who has been appointed an assistant administrator assigned to the Brooklyn center of the New York regional Red Cross blood-donor program. She will supervise administrative and technical operation of borough center at 57 Willoughby St. She is a graduate of Tilden High, Brooklyn College and the Women's Medical College of Pennsylvania. She lives at 1434 Eastern Parkway.

Moe refused to testify and was fired. His friend was promoted to Dean. I stayed with the Red Cross. If they associated me in any way with Moe, they never mentioned it.

Alex Novikoff was also on McCarthy's list. Alex had left Brooklyn College shortly after I graduated in 1944, and had accepted a position at the University of Vermont. They fired him when he was accused by McCarthy of being a communist. He was unemployed for several years, and wrote several books on biology for children. One of the best known, a charming book called *Climbing Our Family Tree*, was about evolution. Alex sent me an autographed copy when it was published. In 1955, when the Albert Einstein College of Medicine was founded in the Bronx, he joined the founding faculty as a pathologist, with the personal endorsement of Albert Einstein. Alex was one of the few members of the initial faculty for whom Einstein personally intervened.

Alex died in 1987. Eric Holzman, chairman of the department of biology at Columbia, was one of the speakers at a memorial service. He had been a student of Alex's, and his reminiscences were very similar to my own memories, but he told a story, possibly apocryphal, of Alex's appearance before the McCarthy committee. It has become part of the Novikoff legend. When he was questioned by Roy Cohen, the lawyer for the committee, about his activities on a certain date, Alex replied cheerfully, "Oh yes, I remember that date well. The acid phosphatase reaction was particularly striking that day. You should have seen the slides!" Alex had many good friends at Columbia, and in 1978, when I was being considered for promotion to full professor, Alex wrote one of the letters of recommendation for me.

Moe also had loyal friends who came to his aid after he was fired. He had been spending summers doing research with Professor Karl Lindegren, the head of microbiology at the University of Southern Illinois in Carbondale. An outspoken conservative Republican, Lindegren called Moe and said, "I know you're a good American and a damn good scientist. This whole Un-American business is nonsense. I've got a place for you in my department if you want it." And so Moe and his family moved to Southern Illinois. I saw them rarely and missed them very much. When Lindegren retired, Moe was made chairman of the department. He developed severe heart disease, had heart surgery at the Rush Presbyterian Hospital in Chicago, and died suddenly during the post-operative period in 1979. It was totally unexpected especially after our relief following the supposedly successful surgery. The worst blizzard of the winter had just ended when we flew out to Chicago for the funeral. It added a nightmarish quality to an already dreadful time: getting plane reservations, and then plowing through Chicago streets still packed with snow, seemed to take forever. My grief at losing my brother, whom I adored, was exceeded only by that of my mother. She had always been a vigorous, cheerful woman and now suddenly seemed old and vulnerable. Losing a beloved child is probably one of the worst disasters that can happen to a parent.

Moe did a lot of research on yeast metabolism and reproduction. His papers were widely published in some of the most prestigious scientific journals. His graduate students became leading figures in biochemistry and microbiology. In the early 1960's he told me how excited he was about a new concept he was working on: the possibility of altering the genetic structure of yeast. He had submitted a preliminary proposal to a journal that had often published his previous research. The proposal was rejected, with a terse letter from the editors. They were surprised that a respected scientist would indulge in that kind of science fiction. It is ironic that the "science fiction" that was scorned a generation ago is the genetic engineering of today. I think it is also a sad commentary on the editors of a leading scientific publication, who did not have the foresight to recognize a new and revolutionary idea. The proposal was published finally in *Perspectives in Biology and Medicine* in the spring of 1969. Its title was "Outline for an Experimental Attack on the Treatment of Certain Varieties of Genetic Disease."

Both Moe and Alex opposed the Korean war. Neither Al nor I were exactly enthusiastic about it, but when he was drafted to go as a physician, he did not hesitate or complain. Taking care of sick and wounded American soldiers was an obligation he felt he owed our country. Many of his letters described a new disease, hemorrhagic fever, that we had not seen before in western countries. It has been with us since.

Al and I wrote to each other daily. He was in a MASH unit, stationed in the bulge of the front lines above the 38th parallel, with hostile North Korean troops on three sides. Mail delivery was erratic and often weeks would go by without a letter. Then a whole batch would arrive in one day. It was an anxious time. Each of his letters assured me that his outfit was being pulled back from the front. I had a map of the area and was adding up the number of miles he said he had withdrawn. It put him somewhere in the middle of the Yellow Sea.

One day his parents phoned me anxiously to tell me that one of their letters to him had been returned unopened. Heart in mouth, I drove to Newark to see the letter myself. Checking the various stamped directions on the envelope, I realized he was in transit back to the United States. Al had served in WW II and apparently that time was credited to him now, decreasing his overseas tour of duty. We didn't know when to expect him and he didn't write to say, hoping to surprise us. Somewhile later, leaving the Red Cross office for lunch, I saw a tall figure in uniform several blocks in front of me. He was striding rapidly in my direction. I knew instantly who it was and broke into a run, oblivious to the stares of witnesses to our reunion.

CHAPTER EIGHT

Marriage

A l and I wished to be married as soon as possible in a small, quiet ceremony. But both his parents and mine had their hearts set on a typical, joyous, Jewish wedding. There is a seven-week period in the Hebrew calendar each spring during which marriages and other festivities can not be performed, except for one day in the middle, called Lag B'Omer. That year, 1952, Lag B'Omer fell on a Sunday, May 25, and synagogues had been booked for weddings and Bar Mitzvahs well in advance. My father and brother scoured the area looking for a place for our wedding and by luck found a synagogue that had not accepted reservations because they were in the process of renovation. Renovations had been completed sooner than expected and so we were the first couple to be married in their shining new hall, with its sparkling chandeliers and blue and gold wall coverings. The wedding canopy under which we were married was a trellis of fresh spring flowers which filled the entire room with their fragrance.

My parents had to go to Schroon Lake to prepare for the summer season and could only return for the weekend of the wedding. Al and I made all the arrangements ourselves and I asked him to help me choose a wedding dress. Neither of us had much experience shopping for fancy clothes and we decided that the occasion demanded a dress from the classiest department store in Manhattan. We walked in like two innocents, holding hands. The saleswomen in the bridal boutique were horrified.

"Don't you know it's bad luck for the groom to see the dress before the wedding?" they cried. They added reluctantly, "Well, if you want to choose a pattern together, it's probably all right. We can have it made up and then your young man wouldn't see the actual dress."

MARRIAGE TO ALVIN J. SCHRAGER, 1952

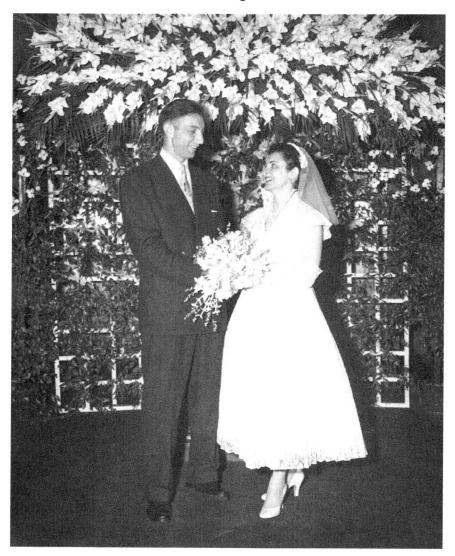

Rising to the occasion with his bizarre sense of humor, Al put his arm around me protectively. "No," he said, solemnly, "We don't have time to have a dress made; we'll have to choose something you have in stock. You see, we have to get married right away." Entering into the spirit, I fluttered my eyelashes and giggled. The good ladies were thoroughly shocked. They were even more unhappy with us when we chose a simple, unconventional dress of ivory lace with a pleated ballet-length skirt, bouffant over a crinoline petticoat. It was one of their least expensive but it fit beautifully, needing no alterations. I was very happy with it and I still have it and it still would fit.

My parents drove in from Schroon Lake on Saturday, the day before the wedding, which was scheduled for the following afternoon. My father had begun to show increasing signs of severe hypertensive cardiovascular disease. These were the years before antihypertensive drugs were available. He had had several "blackouts", periods of unconsciousness. We did not know whether they were TIAs (transient ischemic attacks—small strokes) or cardiac arrhythmias. Neither the Holter heart rhythm monitor nor pacemakers had as yet been invented.

The night before the wedding I was wakened from a restless sleep by my mother calling frantically. I ran to their bedroom and found my father lying on the floor unconscious. Kneeling beside him, I could not find a pulse and he did not seem to be breathing. I started resuscitation, praying desperately, "Dad, please be okay, please." There was a sudden shuddering sigh and he opened his eyes. My mother and I helped him back to bed. I said gently," Dad, I really don't know whether you'll be able to get up for the wedding."

He shook his head, smiling the ironic smile I knew so well. He said in Yiddish, "I will not permit the Angel of Death to interfere with my daughter's wedding day." Several hours later both my parents, smiling proudly, escorted me to the wedding canopy in the joyous Jewish tradition. We told no one about the events of the night before.

Al and I had a very short honeymoon. I had never been in an airplane and Al, having been bounced around Korea in 2-seaters, was not particularly anxious to fly again. We took a train to Miami Beach, sitting up all night in the coach because we couldn't afford a Pullman. But we were blissfully happy and it must have shown. An elderly woman came over to us, unpinning a corsage from her dress.

"My children gave this to me for my birthday. But that's over now, and I can tell you're newlyweds and your life is just beginning. I'd be so happy if you would take it."

I blushed and thanked her. Al muttered to me when she left, "Is it so damn obvious?"

Because of his time in Korea, Al had not completed his training requirements to qualify for specialty boards in Internal Medicine and it was necessary to do this as soon as possible. He accepted a fellowship at Montefiore Hospital in the Bronx. I left my position with the Red Cross in Brooklyn and joined the pediatric practice of the HIP (a group Health Insurance Plan) associated with the hospital. Both Al and I were attracted to the idea of prepaid medical care, and we planned to continue with the group after he completed training requirements. We were quickly disillusioned. Although most of the patients were a pleasure to work with, there was a small but very vocal minority who demanded treatment for the most frivolous reasons because they had paid for it.

As the youngest member of the pediatric staff, I had more than my share of night and weekend calls. I was the only pediatrician in the office on a Christmas weekend, trying to cope with the huge volume of patients. Suddenly the secretary handed me the phone without speaking. Her eyes were wide with fear. A gruff voice said, "I want a house call right away, my daughter is running a fever."

"What is her temperature?" I asked.

"100.2"

"What are her symptoms?"

"Her nose is running and she's beginning to cough."

"It sounds as if she's coming down with a cold. Why don't you—" I got no further.

"Listen, sister," he barked. "Do you know who I am?" He identified himself as the president of a large union, all of whose members were registered with Montefiore's HIP. "You'd better get your ass down here on the double if you know what's good for you."

"Oh, really?" I snapped back. "Well, do you know who I am? I'm not your sister, I'm the only doctor on call here today, and I have an office full of patients a lot sicker than your daughter. Now, if you insist on having her seen, you can bring her down, wait your turn and I'll examine her. But I will not come out on a house call." He slammed down the receiver.

I learned later that he had lodged a complaint against me with the then-Mayor Impelliteri and there had been a full-scale investigation. I only found out about it several months after the event when it came up for discussion at a medical staff business meeting. I was angry that no one had told me or given me the chance to defend myself. They assured me that the investigation had proven the complaint unjustified and they saw no reason to trouble me. I was somewhat mollified, but both Al and I had the distinct feeling this was not a system we would enjoy.

We had rented a studio apartment some distance from the hospital. Rentals were scarce and expensive and we felt very fortunate to find this one on Muliner Avenue, close to the Bronx Zoo and the Botanical Gardens. It was a pleasant area and we enjoyed long walks through the zoo and gardens when we had time off together. We had to commute to the hospital and that posed some problems. I had bought a car with my earnings from the Red Cross. It was a brand new Plymouth and I was very proud of it. But we both needed a car. We had different schedules and couldn't always travel to the hospital together. Al was occasionally on call for emergencies at night. I had to make house calls daily, as well as go to the office. We couldn't afford two cars and even if we could, Al had never learned to drive. I had been driving since I was sixteen, when we lived at Schroon Lake. I had taken my driving test in Ticonderoga, where the examiner had threatened to flunk me because I was riding the clutch on a hill instead of using the brake. There were no automatic transmissions in those days.

I tried to give Al driving lessons. There is no surer way of destroying a marriage. By mutual consent, he registered in a driving school after the first two attempts. We continued to struggle along with one car after Al got his license, trusting to luck that we would never have two emergencies at the same time. Providence must have been with us because we survived the year without mishap.

I set about organizing a home that observed the dietary laws of Judaism, as I had promised. I had distinct memories of the kosher home my mother had kept when her parents had lived with us before we moved to Schroon Lake. I felt confident that it would be no problem establishing one again but it was a bit more difficult than I had anticipated. Al's family had traditions that were different from my family. As an example, we had to keep meat and dairy dishes and utensils separate. My family labeled all things related to meat with a red symbol and all dairy things blue. Al's family did just the opposite. Since my family no longer kept kosher I had to adapt to his way. It was very confusing. I later learned that my family's way was the one generally accepted and to this day our friends who observe dietary laws become quite disturbed when they see the reversal of colors in my kitchen.

Although Al's family kept the dietary laws, they were not strictly observant in other matters, such as riding on the Sabbath. They rarely attended synagogue except for the major holidays. Al became much more observant after his father's death, which occurred a little less than two years after our marriage. He observed the eleven-month period of mourning very strictly, saying Kaddish, prayers for the dead, in synagogue twice daily. He wanted a stricter observance of the Sabbath and other aspects of Jewish law at home. This was not what we had agreed on, and initially I resented it. But many compromises had to be made in our marriage. If I were to practice medicine and raise a family, I needed the wholehearted support of my husband, and Al was ready to give it to me despite his initial reservations about careers for women. To please him, I was ready to keep a more religious home.

I also recognized that religious observance established the unequivocal identity of our children and what was expected of them. Because of my strange childhood I felt that I had never been part of any group—not in the city, and not in Schroon Lake. Those feelings of alienation are with me to this day, although much modified by loving family and friends. I was happy that I could raise children who were proud and comfortable with their identity.

CHAPTER NINE

Combining Private Practice
with Raising a Family

After finishing his training at the end of 1953, Al was offered a position doing oncology research at Yale on the recommendation of one of his mentors at Montefiore. I often wondered what our life would have been like if he had accepted, which I urged him to do. But he felt the need to make a decent living and to be close to his parents. We looked for a place to open a practice. Al wanted to settle in Newark but I never liked city life and there was a mass migration to the suburbs from that city. We considered several outlying areas that seemed to be growing rapidly due to the migration from Newark. Al had several friends who had moved from Newark to these suburbs. One of these owned a professional building and had an office suite to rent. He was a little man with a quick, nervous manner and a fixed smile that showed all his teeth and the gold fillings in back. He was effusive in his joy that a good ol' pal was moving into the area. We had just about concluded an agreement to rent the office when he learned that I would be practicing there as well as Al.

"I didn't know your wife was a doctor," he said. "If both of you are going to use the office, the rent is doubled."

"But we're paying you for exclusive use of that office space," Al argued. "I don't see why the rent should be increased because both of us use it."

"Two doctors, two rents," he replied.

Al started to argue again, but I turned toward the door. "I've changed my mind. I wouldn't practice here no matter what the rent is. I don't like the atmosphere."

We looked at several other suburbs around Newark—Milburn, Maplewood, Livingston, Short Hills. They were expanding rapidly and it seemed obvious that they would need more doctors. We decided to seek advice from physicians practicing in the area. Their response was always the same: "We have too many doctors here already. You'd better look elsewhere."

One day we were cruising through an unfamiliar area south of Newark. We got lost and were on a small secondary road we had never seen before. The area seemed more rural than the suburbs we had visited. We entered a picturesque little town with a small lake in the center. A beautiful white church stood next to the lake, reflected in its waters. Swans were gliding majestically on its surface.

"This town is lovely," I said. "What is its name?"

Al didn't know, and we stopped to ask a passerby. "This is Westfield", he said.

Al said, "Never heard of it."

I said, "Let's park and explore a bit."

We wandered around the central business area. Many of the buildings were constructed of red brick in a colonial style that reminded me of Williamsburg. Walking a short distance, we came to a synagogue with similar Georgian architecture, blending with the colonial appearance of the town. (To my regret the synagogue was modernized with entirely different architecture when it was enlarged several years later.) The peace and tranquility of this lovely town brought back memories of Schroon Lake.

"This is it!" I cried. "This is where I want to live and raise children!"

Most of our peers were doing extensive demographic research and consulting with practice management experts to find the right place to set up practice. My reasons for choosing Westfield would not have met with their approval. We knew no one, had no professional connections. Al was more than a little reluctant, but gamely went about looking for an office to rent. He found one and said philosophically, "Well, if we starve here we can always eat the swans."

Our office was situated in a converted house owned by a group of obstetricians. They practiced in offices on the first floor, we on the second. They were cordial and encouraging and the rent was fair but they did not refer many patients to us. Our start in practice was extremely slow, complicated by the terminal illness of Al's father. He needed repeated hospitalizations and Al was with him continually. This made him unavailable to see patients on a regular basis. I made some income covering the practice of other pediatricians when they took time off.

After his father's death, Al got a part-time job with the V.A. His private practice began to grow and gradually things improved for both of us. Dr. Daniel Hackett, one of the town's leading pediatricians, had just ended his partnership with several other pediatricians, and asked me to help cover his practice. He was getting older and wanted to cut down on the hours he was available to see patients, so I became very busy.

One evening I was called to see one of his patients whose parents lived in the most affluent part of town. The door was answered by a maid who whispered she would accompany me to the child's bedroom. The mother had left word that she did not want to be disturbed. She was meeting with friends in the large, luxurious living room just to the left of the central hall with its gracefully curving staircase.

When I examined the lovely little four-year-old, his tousled blond hair wet with perspiration from a high fever, I noted he had a bad cough and seemed a bit short of breath. I could hear the sounds of pneumonia in his right lung. He kept crying for his mommy and I reassured him that she was just downstairs and I was going to speak with her immediately so we could start medicine to get him better. He seemed comforted, sniffed and nodded. Although I thought he would respond to treatment at home, I was concerned that if he did not improve rapidly we would have to consider hospitalization. I told the maid I had to speak with the mother. While I stood in the hall writing some prescriptions, I could hear the meeting in the next room. Apparently they were a group of graduates from a prestigious woman's college being addressed by a member of the faculty. Through the open archway leading to the living room I could see the speaker. He was a tall, tweedy man of middle age with iron-gray hair. He stood leaning casually by the fireplace, gesturing expansively with pipe in one hand. A dozen or so alumnae were seated on the beautifully upholstered silk damask armchairs and sofa, listening with rapt attention.

"You have all had a wonderful education," he said. "You should have the right to continue with careers of your own. You don't all have to be housewives."

The mother finally appeared. She was a slim blonde woman, hair stylishly set, elegant suit in perfect harmony with her surroundings. Her blue eyes glinted coldly. She was obviously angry at being interrupted. I explained my concerns and tried to be reassuring but told her hospitalization might be necessary if the child did not improve with the medication I had prescribed. "Yes, we'll see," she said abruptly, then added, "the next time Dr. Hackett is away, if we call you, I expect you to use the servant's entrance."

"The next time Dr. Hackett is away, call a different pediatrician," I retorted. "I don't use the servant's entrance." I thought it ironic that in the midst of a meeting on the rights of women to have careers she reduced the status of a woman with a career to that of a servant. I was sure she had never spoken to Dr. Hackett that way.

As our practices began to improve, I became pregnant. Several weeks before my due date I was scheduled to take a series of examinations, given annually by the American Board of Pediatrics to qualify as a Board-certified pediatrician. The exams were given at a large university center and were in two parts; a very intensive written exam that occupied all of the first day and then oral exams on the following day. The orals were conducted by some of the most noted pediatricians in the country. My first examiner, the author of a well-known pediatric textbook, looked with obvious disapproval at my far-advanced pregnancy.

"Young woman" he said, "Do you seriously intend to practice after the birth of your baby?"

I attempted some half-hearted humor. "Do you seriously think I would be taking these exams if I didn't intend to continue?" I said.

He grunted. "Are you using your maiden name or your husband's?" he asked.

"I'm using my husband's name," I answered.

"Good" he replied. "If you were using your maiden name, I would flunk you on the spot."

We named our first-born son Lewis, in memory of Al's father. Because that memory was so fresh, Al's family had difficulty calling the little baby by the same name and we called him Luke. To this day you can identify how long people know him by whether they call him Lew or Luke. He was born on July 21, 1955 at St. Barnabas Hospital in Newark. We had joined St. Barnabas as soon as we set up practice because the obstetricians in our building used it as their main referring hospital. One of them, Dr. Jessie Read, was my obstetrician. She, Al, and some of the other doctors we knew crowded into the labor room to visit when I was admitted.

They were having a grand time socializing while my contractions were getting closer and closer together. "Hey guys," I said, "will you get the hell out of here. I've got work to do. I think the baby is coming soon."

"Nah," said Jessie, "You don't look ornery enough." But they left.

Less than an hour later, I shrieked, "The baby's coming!"

Jessie ran back in, took one look and rushed me to the delivery room, where the baby was born within minutes. It was natural childbirth in its most basic form.

It was the custom to keep women hospitalized and in bed for a full week after delivery. The hospital was not air-conditioned, and we were in the middle of a heat wave. I awoke early the next morning feeling very hot and uncomfortable. Without giving it a second thought, I got out of bed to shower. The nurse came in, found the bed empty and became greatly alarmed.

"I'm in here," I called from the shower.

They were very annoyed with me, and the head of nursing came in to tell me that even doctors had to obey the rules. I was appropriately apologetic.

I returned to practice less than a week after I was released from the hospital. I tried to organize my schedule around breast feeding but it was very difficult and I could not continue for very long. I still kept running home several times during the day to the apartment we had rented in Cranford, a neighboring community. (There were very few apartments to rent in Westfield.) Clara Wiener, a motherly German woman, helped me care for the baby. She was very devoted and stayed with us for over twenty years. At first we couldn't afford her full-time and Al and I had to arrange our schedules so that there would always be someone to care for the baby. There were times when I had an emergency and would take Luke with me to the hospital, to the office, or on a house call. When I look back now at the way we had to cope, I shudder.

We joined Overlook Hospital in Summit in 1954, although we continued to use St. Barnabas as our main hospital until they moved to Livingston. Overlook was closer than St. Barnabas, and when St. Barnabas moved to Livingston it was even more inconvenient. Many of the doctors for whom we covered used Overlook exclusively. At that time it was only a modest community hospital. The staff was small and we all knew each other by name. I was the only woman in the pediatrics department and I received a courteous but cool reception from the other doctors. At first, I had few patients to hospitalize, but I attended all conferences, silent but observant. As I became more at ease I began to venture a few questions or suggestions about the diagnosis or treatment of patients being discussed. These comments were usually ignored, but I noted that frequently another member of the department would repeat what I had said and then they would be acted on.

Not long after I joined the staff I hospitalized a critically ill little girl with a ruptured appendix. Her mother was in near-hysteria, and I suggested that we go for a cup of coffee and a quiet talk while the child was in the operating room. The coffee shop was crowded and noisy, but in the back was a quiet alcove where several tables were reserved for doctors. As we went to sit down there, a waitress bustled up and said officiously, "I'm sorry, this area is for doctors only."

"I'm Dr. Schrager" I said, showing her my identification. "I've recently joined the pediatric attending staff."

She sniffed disapprovingly. "We're not used to seating women back here."

I smiled at her icily. "Well, you'd better get used to it," I told her.

Regrettably, in those early days I found that some of the greatest resistance to my acceptance as a doctor came from other women. An assistant nursing director was particularly cold and unfriendly. An obese woman with double chins and a perpetual scowl, she stalked the corridors with an air of unquestioned authority that struck terror into the hearts of the younger nurses. Even the doctors treated her with great deference.

One day, a patient of Al's was admitted as an emergency to the Intensive Care Unit. A surgeon was going to see him in consultation but Al was anxious to get up to the hospital as soon as possible. He had an office full of sick patients and he chafed at the delay. "Look," I said, "I know that family well. I take care of their kids. I'm on my way to the hospital and can look in on the father and check what's going on."

Al was greatly relieved. "Call me as soon as you see him." I agreed and went directly to the ICU. I reviewed the man's medical chart, examined him and began to discuss his condition and our management plans with him and his wife. They were very grateful I had come so promptly and seemed reassured by our talk. The assistant nursing director suddenly burst into the room, snatched the chart from my hands and exclaimed, "You have no right to look at this. And visitors are restricted to immediate family. Leave immediately!"

I said quietly, "Perhaps we can discuss this elsewhere." We went to the conference room behind the nurse's station. I closed the door. Shaking with fury, it was one of the few times I ever raised my voice in the hospital. "HOW DARE YOU! How dare you behave so unprofessionally in front of a patient!" She paled, and said defensively, "But you have no right to be on this floor."

"Since when are a doctor's privileges in this hospital restricted to a specific floor? I'm covering for my husband, just as many other doctors cover for their partners. When have you ever prevented any doctor from examining a pediatric patient? If you ever interfere with me again, I'm going to lodge a formal complaint with the administration."

I never had difficulty with her again. I went back to see the patient and his wife who had been upset by the encounter. I said, "It's okay. She just didn't realize I was a doctor."

I will never forget a neonatal emergency I had at about that time. An infant was born with a depressed skull fracture, so severe that the whole side of her skull was indented and her features were distorted. Accepted treatment was a neurosurgical procedure to raise the depression with a hook. I called frantically for the neurosurgeon, Dr. Henry Liss, and finally located him. "I'm in the middle of an operation that's going to take about four hours," he said. "I'll get down to the nursery as soon as I can."

There was no other neurosurgeon on our staff and I became desperate, fearing the delay might cause brain damage. Suddenly the idea occurred to me to raise the depression by suction and I realized that a hand breast pump would just about cover the depressed area. I called Henry back and asked if there would be any contraindication to attempting this procedure. He laughed. "Go ahead and try—I don't think it will work, but you can't do any damage."

I applied suction with a breast pump but air leakage occurred and I was unsuccessful. Grimly, I decided to coat the edges of the rubber pump with vaseline to obtain a tighter seal. There was a sudden pop! and the entire area raised up. The infant's features returned to normal. She was a lovely little girl.

When Henry Liss examined the baby, he was amazed. "If I hadn't seen the X-rays you took before and after, I wouldn't have believed it."

We decided to report this procedure in the pediatric literature and it was accepted for publication. The article was chosen for inclusion in the 1972 Yearbook of Pediatrics, which summarizes the significant advances of the year. More importantly, the grateful father, a football coach at West Point, got us tickets to sit on the 50 yard line with all the uniformed brass. That Christmas I gave Henry Liss a present—a breast pump to add to his neurosurgical equipment.

The hospital was in a state of transition between 1955 and 1970. It was growing rapidly as the surrounding suburbs grew. Young doctors, most of them the product of excellent medical schools and years of postgraduate training, were attracted to the area. A small community hospital could not satisfy their needs.

They wanted the support of a local hospital that had a resident staff on call twenty-four hours a day and that employed full-time radiologists, anesthesiologists, pathologists—well-trained hospital-based specialists who knew the rapid medical progress of the second half of the twentieth century. In short they wanted a teaching hospital affiliated with a medical school.

During this time a heated controversy developed between the Old Guard and the Young Turks. We had an elected Chief of Pediatrics who served for two years with the option of re-election for another two years. This position rotated among the three senior members of the department, who opposed any change. The younger members wanted new blood, but were not ready to bleed themselves. Opposition to the status quo could cause financial and other problems involving patient referrals. Initially I was uninvolved. I was pregnant with my second child and taking care of a home, a two-year-old, and a practice occupied all my time.

I gave birth to my second son, Ralph, on July 12, 1957. As with Luke, I took off minimal time during pregnancy and after his birth. This is not something I would recommend or be proud of. It was simply the way women in medicine practiced during those years. We felt we had to continually prove ourselves equal to the men.

The night before his birth I was called to see a newborn in respiratory distress. I rushed to the hospital and entered through the emergency department because all other entrances were locked at night.

"Just a minute, mother," one of the nurses called. "We'll take you up by wheelchair."

Drawing myself up with as much dignity as my altered form and waddling gait would allow, I responded, "I'm not in labor. I'm Dr. Schrager and I've been called to see a sick newborn."

They stared at me in astonishment and disbelief. Two days later the infant I had resuscitated and my baby were lying next to eachother in the same nursery.

I stayed in the hospital for the customary eight days, until after the ritual circumcision, as I had done with Luke. My parents, some relatives, and many of the doctors and nurses came to the Brit Milah which we celebrated with the usual drinks and delicacies. I had not gained much weight during my pregnancy and had dressed for the occasion in high heels and a pretty summer dress with flared skirt that I had worn before becoming pregnant. After the ceremony they put me in a wheelchair holding the baby in preparation for wheeling me out of the hospital. In the elevator I noted that my father had become very short of breath. With his severe heart disease, the exertion and excitement were more than he could tolerate.

"Dad," I said, "You sit in the wheelchair and hold the baby. I can stand."

Several doctors and nurses entered the elevator on a lower floor. They looked with consternation at the elderly man in the wheelchair with the baby. "Where is the mother?" they asked. Everyone laughed when I held up my hand.

We had begun to make a respectable living in private practice and in 1958 we built a house with office attached. Maintaining an office in the house was financially daunting. When we had the plans drawn we had been strongly advised to provide for adequate office space in excess of our present needs. It made sense but we had very little money to spare. We decided to take out a huge mortgage.

My father nodded his approval. He was almost completely bed-ridden by this time, but he was still alert and excited by the idea that we would have our own home at last. "You know I hate to borrow money," he said. "The only exception is to buy land to live on, or for business."

He insisted on lending us the money for a downpayment. My parents had sold the property at Schroon Lake a few years before when it became obvious that they could no longer manage the business, and that money was now available to us. He was happy that we were not trying to economize but were building properly, for the future. We took him to see the house shortly before it was completed. He had difficulty walking but Al and I supported him on either side. I realized that my stalwart, stoic father had become more emotional with age but it was still upsetting to see the tears rolling down his sunken cheeks. "It is good," he whispered. "It is very good. I am glad that the money from Schroon Lake helped you build this beautiful house." My father died a few weeks after we moved in.

The house was built on several different levels so that the living quarters were totally separate from the offices. A door in the kitchen led down to the offices. In addition to a large waiting room and four examining rooms at street level, we used part of the basement for a lead-lined X-ray room and a laboratory. During the Cuban missile crisis in1963 I stocked soft drinks, crackers and peanut butter and jelly in a closet in that lead-lined room. It seems ludicrous now but during that time many families were building bomb shelters in their back yards and the media were debating the ethics of shooting neighbors who wanted to invade your shelter during a nuclear attack.

Both children attended the public schools in Westfield, which are excellent. Their elementary school, Jefferson, is just a few short blocks from us. Luke insisted on walking there himself after the first few days of kindergarten, and when Ralph started school two years later, they went off together without assistance. As small children, Luke and Ralph seemed to accept our busy household as normal family living. Luke, two years older, was very protective of his baby brother. He bossed him around unmercifully, but Ralph good-naturedly accepted it without complaint. It was obvious that they were very fond of each other. Once, Luke snatched Ralph out of the path of a car that had backed into our driveway to turn around.

Ralph was particularly fun-loving and mischievous. As soon as he could walk, he would head for the street. Al would pick him up and remonstrate, but as soon as he was put down he was on his way again, laughing at our discomfiture. Al finally lost patience and gave his bottom a resounding smack. He didn't realize that Ralph had a very full diaper. Little pieces flew out in all directions. Al turned to me with an apologetic grin. "Glor," he said, "I just beat the shit out of your son!"

When Luke was in kindergarten, someone brought a litter of baby kittens to school and offered to give them away. Luke immediately bonded with a tiny black and white furball. And so Blackie came to live with us. She grew into a very strange cat. She was not at all affectionate, and accepted petting for only short periods of time. One had the feeling that she owned the premises and tolerated our

OUR SONS' CHILDHOOD IN WESTFIELD

1957   **1960**

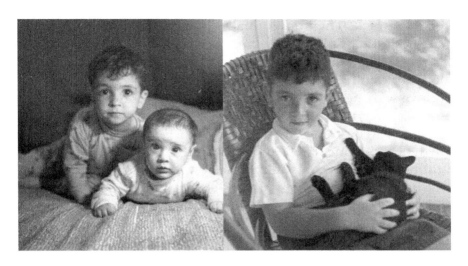

1961   **1968**

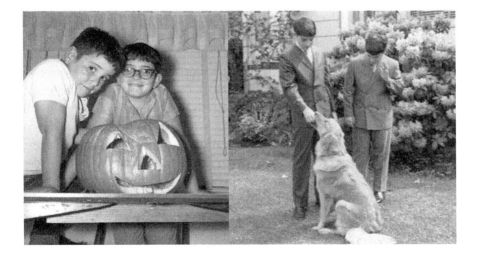

presence as noblesse oblige. At 3:00 PM every school day, she would disappear and go down to the school, four blocks away, to meet the boys. She would not greet them, purring, but would just turn tail and walk back home, glancing over her shoulder to be sure they were following. Occasionally, she would disappear into the bushes, stalk them stealthily, and suddenly pounce out for the attack. They would make appropriate noises of terror. Satisfied, she would resume her march, tail twitching.

The boys wanted to have a dog as well. One of our patients had a golden retriever, at that time a very rare breed, and we fell in love with her. We heard of a kennel in Mystic, Connecticut that was offering retriever puppies for sale, and made a special trip there to buy one. We named her Misty after the place of her birth. I was concerned about Blackie's reaction to this new addition, but it was needless. Blackie was not at all afraid of this playful puppy, much larger than she was. She seemed to tolerate her as one would a mischievous child. If Misty became too annoying, she would swat her across the nose, but never with her claws out.

Misty was as affectionate as Blackie was not. We decided to have her bred so that we could let the boys see the birth of a litter of puppies. We arrived somewhat early for our appointment at the kennels, and found that the breeder was also a dog trainer. He hurried over to us, wearing padded vest, gauntlets and face mask, and warned us to stay in the car, windows raised, until he had finished his session training a group of guard dogs. It was the time of the Newark riots, and there were occasional acts of violence in the usually peaceful suburbs that surrounded us. I was still making housecalls, day and night, and thought it advisable to have Misty trained in some elementary guard dog procedures, since she always accompanied me in the car. As soon as the trainer was free, I spoke to him about it. He looked disparagingly at Misty, who was happily wagging her tail. "The only way that dog would hurt anyone," he said, "is if she licked him to death." Unfortunately, the breeding was unsuccessful and we didn't try again

The 1960's were a turbulent period. In addition to the Newark riots, drug use, particularly LSD, was common. The police were often called out to see someone who had a "bad trip" and was hallucinating. Unlike other doctors, we could always be found, and we spent many nights talking down a frantic patient. One of us would sometimes go upstairs to check on the children and we would find them with their noses pressed against the window, staring down at the police cars with their lights flashing, and the commotion in the street.

One of my patients who had a "bad trip" was an adolescent girl who was an excellent student. This was her first experience with drugs. She had been at a party with a new boyfriend whom she wanted to impress. Her hallucinations would have been funny if they weren't so sad. She kept writing at an imaginary typewriter, her fingers flying over the "keyboard" as she "typed." She was in a panic, screaming, "The words are disappearing! The typewriter is broken! I'll never finish this paper! I'll flunk out!"

One night, when Al was out on an emergency at the hospital, the police came to the door to ask me to examine a child who was having a convulsion in a nearby house. Paramedics and 911 were not yet in existence. "I'll be glad to go, but I can't leave the children alone," I said. And so the boys had a cop as volunteer babysitter.

Al and I were so involved with practice and the constant care of our parents that we had little time to attend our sons' extracurricular activities, such as Little League, wrestling matches, and orchestra. When Luke was in the sixth grade, he was chosen to play Scrooge in Dickens Christmas Carol. I happened to see his teacher at the supermarket a few days before the performance and she told me how nervous she was. "He has to memorize so much and he's on stage constantly," she said. "But he's such a good student, I'm sure he'll do fine. Besides, you've probably been rehearsing with him daily!" I nodded weakly. Not only had I not rehearsed with him, I hadn't even checked to see if he had been learning the part by himself.

Totally guilt-ridden, I went home to speak with him. "Don't worry, Mom," he said, "I know my lines." The play was a great success and when it was over we went to a local Howard Johnson's for ice cream. The place was packed with students and parents who had seen the show. When we entered, they rose and began to applaud. It was a memorable experience but I had the uncomfortable feeling that Al and I were basking in reflected glory that we did not deserve.

Our house was the center for holiday celebrations—New Year's, Thanksgiving, the Jewish High Holidays, Passover. On one of these occasions (I've forgotten which) I was busy in the kitchen preparing dinner, concentrating on my matzoh balls which require a delicate touch to make them light and fluffy. I was particularly proud of mine, the sign of a good Jewish cook, and the family wouldn't consider any festive meal complete if I didn't serve them with my home-made chicken soup. The boys were playing with their cousins on the top floor of the house. That long room is now our library, but was then a spare bedroom and playroom. Suddenly we heard a loud crash and the sound of breaking glass. We ran up to find Ralph covered with blood. He had thrown a basketball which had broken the ceiling light fixture. He had been looking up and the falling glass had neatly bisected his face from forehead to chin.

Al carried him down to the office and we tried to stop the bleeding. I looked at Al desperately. I often sewed up small lacerations in children, but this was more than I could handle. We were reluctant to take him to an emergency room, and the chances of locating a plastic surgeon on a holiday weekend were remote. When we finally had the bleeding controlled and cleansed his face, we realized that the lacerations were extensive but superficial. We decided to pull the cut edges of skin together with steri-strips, small bits of adhesive.

Luke critically eyed the line of tapes down the middle of Ralph's face. They extended from hairline to chin. He said, "you look like Frankenstein."

Al said, "Do you feel okay now, Ralph?"

Ralph said, "Sure. Gee, I'm glad you didn't have to take me to a *real* doctor!" The cuts healed without a scar except for a small one on his upper lip.

Neither of our sons seemed particularly impressed with their parents' profession. One evening at dinner, Luke said, "Everyone asks me what I want to be when I grow up. I don't know what I want to be, but I know what I don't want to be. I don't want to be a doctor!" "Me, neither!" said Ralph. Luke looked at us with a puzzled and vulnerable expression. "But what else *is* there?" he asked. Al and I were amused but also somewhat sad. We felt that our professional lives had influenced our sons more than we would have wished.

We knew we would be sacrificing privacy when we built house and office in one building but these disturbances didn't happen very often. Dinner was occasionally interrupted by anxious patients who rang the front door bell after hours. Al was philosophic about it. "If they had telephoned, and the office was somewhere else, we probably would have to run there or go on a house call to see them anyway—like this, we only have to go downstairs."

We had seriously considered the advantages and disadvantages. Many people had discouraged us from having house and office together and compared it to "Mom and Pop living above the store." But we felt that being close to the children would be worth it. We never regretted it.

Although we had little free time to spend with the boys during the school year, we always vacationed together during the summer and winter holidays. True to our usual habit of not following the crowds, we went north in the winter, to the less-busy ski resorts and south in the summer, to Hilton Head or Florida.

Al and I were moderately competent skiers but the boys soon outclassed us. One afternoon we saw a child take a spectacular fall, doing a somersault in the air and landing in a snowdrift. He got up and began brushing off the snow, but he was still unrecognizable. We thought the boys were skiing on a different slope, and I said to Al, "Thank Heavens that wasn't one of our kids." A short time later, I was on the line for the ski lift when the Abominable Snowman came skiing up to me. It said proudly, "Hi, Mom. Did you see the tumble I took?" "It" was Ralph.

In the summer we played tennis, swam, and water skied. The first time we took the children water skiing we had a surly instructor who had no patience with them. He gave them a few muttered instructions and told Luke, "You're first. Get in the water and put on your skis." The instructor started the boat with a jerk, expecting him to fall on his face. On his first attempt, Luke got right to his feet and began to ski. He shouted to the instructor, "You mean like this?"

"Yeah," muttered the instructor, "like that."

One Passover holiday, good friends convinced us to spend the week with them at a large hotel. It had been a stressful year and I was particularly grateful not to have the exhausting task of preparing the house for the holiday. The hotel had a large indoor pool and my daily swim was an added bonus. On the last day we packed early and I realized I had time for a swim before we checked out. I was peacefully doing my laps when a sudden commotion drew my attention. They were pulling the inert body of a small boy from the bottom of the pool. Dripping wet, I dashed over and found that the life guard was just starting resuscitation.

CPR as we know it today was being taught in medical centers but was not as yet standard procedure. The lifeguard was using an antiquated, ineffective method. He looked up at me and said soothingly, "Don't worry, mother, I'm taking care of your little boy. He'll be okay."

I said, "I am not his mother, I 'm a doctor and he won't be okay if you continue what you're doing. You'd better learn CPR! Get out of my way!" I pushed him aside and began mouth-to-mouth resuscitation and cardiac massage. After an eternity the child coughed, vomited up a lot of water, and began to cry. The boy's father and the house physician arrived. The doctor put his stethoscope to the boy's chest. The father asked anxiously, "Will he be alright, doc?" The doctor nodded. The father grabbed his hands and said fervently, "Thanks, doc. You saved my boy's life." Unnoticed, I silently slipped away.

When I told Al what had happened, he thought it important that the management know and take steps to train the lifeguards in CPR. I went to the front desk and asked to speak to the manager. They said he wasn't available but I could speak to the head of security. I found him in his office, sitting under a huge portrait of J. Edgar Hoover. With his bulging eyes and pot belly, there was a pronounced resemblance between the two. He was unimpressed by my story and said dismissively, "This hotel has been in business fifty years and we haven't had a drowning yet."

"Well, you almost had one today," I said and left.

We took the boys camping through the national parks one summer. We toured Yellowstone, Bryce, Zion, and the north rim of the Grand Canyon, cooked over a campfire or camp stove, and slept under the stars in makeshift tents and sleeping blankets. We all loved it. Each morning, Al would rise very early to say his morning prayers. He would hike a distance from the campsite to have privacy as he put on tallis, the prayer shawl, and tfillin, the Jewish phylacteries worn for prayer. One morning he found a small clearing in the forest, quiet and deserted. As he was finishing his prayers, removing the leather thongs from his left arm, he became aware of an elderly woman who was watching him intently from the edge of the clearing. Dressed in tweeds and stout shoes and carrying a walking stick, she came up to him and said with typical British directness, "What were you doing?"

"I was praying," said Al.

"Yes, I deduced as much, but what religion are you?"

Folding his arms gravely, Al said, "I am of the tribe of the Blue Heron. We never made peace with the white man. I say Indian prayers."

"But what were you praying for?" asked the lady.

"I pray for rain," said Al.

"But my good man, it rarely rains here this time of year," said the lady.

"That is why I pray," said Al.

He came back to camp and told us of his adventure and we laughed as we packed our gear into the car and headed out. We weren't on the road a half hour when, with frightening speed and suddenness, a violent storm hit. The rain poured, the thunder echoed off the mountains, bolts of lightening flashed across the sky. Luke leaned forward from the back seat and shouted above the din, "Dad, I bet that English lady is pretty impressed."

Our holidays were short and infrequent because our practices were becoming increasingly busy. Theoretically we were beginning to make a good income but actually there was little money left for luxuries. As the "wealthy doctors" of the family we were often approached for loans which Al would never refuse. Most were paid back as soon as possible but Al had one cousin who borrowed repeatedly without ever indicating when the money would be returned. When he asked for money the third or fourth time and we learned he was going to use it to take his family to Spain for the summer I rebelled. It was the first loan Al ever refused. We never heard from that cousin again.

Other events were making life at home less than idyllic. In the middle sixties Al's mother began developing signs of Alzheimer's disease. She refused to leave her home in Newark even though it became increasingly obvious that she was having difficulty living by herself. She became increasingly agitated when we suggested that we would find a companion to live with her. "No! I will not have a stranger living in my house!"

Al, always a devoted son, went in twice a day to bring her food and take care of her needs. It was the time of the Newark riots and her home was in the middle of the violence. The whole area was cordoned off by the police. Entrance was limited to residents but the police allowed Al his frequent visits. I lived in constant fear for his safety.

Between his absorption with his patients and his mother's care, he had little free time for his family. It was taking its toll on our marriage and on our children. When they were smaller, he would often play with them and join their football games on the back lawn. Now he was preoccupied and was never available for such play. I resented the fact that his priorities appeared to put his mother above his wife and children, and we began to have some of the stormy sessions that had characterized our courtship. After one particularly heated argument, I sobbed, "If you mother and I fell overboard, I wonder which one of us you would rescue first." With his quizzical, half-amused look, Al said, "My mother, of course. She can't swim and you're an expert. You would probably end up saving both of us." I glared at him, and then burst out laughing, struck by the ludicrous spectacle that would make.

As his mother's condition deteriorated, she became increasingly confused and disoriented and it was impossible for her to live alone. Al would not consider sending her to a nursing home and so she came to live with us. We had to employ a full-time nurse to care for her. She had to be watched carefully.

In addition, our home had become a haven for other family members in distress. My mother, a fiercely independent woman, had been living in a retirement village since the death of my father. She developed severe osteoporosis which led to multiple compression fractures of her vertebrae. Despite this, she insisted on staying home unless the pain became too severe, when she would come to us until she was again able to manage on her own. There were times when we had both mothers in residence. My mother was greatly troubled by the strain this was putting on our marriage and our children. An outspoken woman, she expressed her concerns openly. That only increased family frictions. I felt caught in the middle. I understood my mother's distress at our disrupted family life, but I also understood Al's reluctance to place his mother in a nursing home. He visited patients in nursing homes every day and knew every institution in the area. Nursing homes have improved recently but in those days they were all unpleasant places, smelling of urine and strong disinfectant. There was no easy solution to our problem.

We also harbored other relatives in times of crisis. Al's aunt, who lived in Pittsburgh, came to stay with us when her husband died. She was destitute but very unhappy being away from her circle of friends. We solved that problem by finding her an apartment in Pittsburgh and supporting her there for many years.

The number of elderly, unhappy people living with us sometimes seemed overwhelming. We were supporting two mothers, an aunt, a full-time elderly LPN for Al's mother, and Clara, who was also getting on in years. Clara did most of the housekeeping but little of the cooking. She was an uninspired cook and whenever possible I prepared the meals, particularly for the Sabbath. I wouldn't recommend our daily menu. It often consisted of leftovers. There were no kosher take-out meals except for delicatessen which we used sparingly for special occasions.

In addition our expenses included the salaries of the office staff—a receptionist and two nurses, Noreen Rouillard, Barbara

Hermitt and Marcie Raney. Later, Gloria Krempa joined the staff. They were all excellent help and we enjoyed working together. They stayed with us for many years, and became good friends. The office environment was very pleasant. The staff got to know most of our patients and their families by their first names. When patients called and asked for Dr. Schrager there was confusion at first about which one they wanted. Staff and patients solved the problem spontaneously. They called us Dr. Al and Dr. Gloria. I winced when I first heard the term. It sounded so tacky, like a Grade B movie. But I soon got used to it and realized it was a practical solution to the problem. To this day I still meet former patients who call me Dr. Gloria.

I instituted another tradition. Our full-time staff was often too busy to take care of the routine tasks such as filing, and I decided to hire a high school senior who could help them. I chose a young girl who was a patient and who had shown some interest in becoming a doctor. I thought that exposing a young woman to the practice of a woman doctor might influence her to choose the same career. When she graduated and left for college, she recommended another girl just entering her senior year. This chain continued unbroken for many years. Several did become doctors.

CHAPTER TEN

Chief of Pediatrics

The hospital was expanding, and without being consciously aware of it I was becoming more involved in organizing improvements in pediatrics. A member of the pediatric staff, Dr. Arnold Constad, was a founding member of Physicians for Automotive Safety, along with Dr. Seymour Charles. The organization tried to educate parents that infants should have appropriate restraints in cars from the moment they left the hospital on their first ride home. Many doctors and nurses scoffed at the idea, and Arnold and I launched a full-scale campaign to make infant seats available for sale in the hospital gift shop. We also organized a program that would teach automotive safety to new mothers. We were one of the first hospitals in the U.S. to institute such a service. Inadvertently, I found myself increasingly involved in the discussions to modernize the pediatric department. When the Young Turks asked me to run for chief in 1970, I agreed and to my amazement I was elected.

Being chief gave one a certain amount of prestige, but it was a thankless job. There was no money involved: the honor was considered adequate. One had to settle disputes between various members of the department or between our department and others. These often involved controversies about who was in charge when several doctors were on the same case. All members of the medical staff had a host of responsibilities unrelated to their private practices. They had to attend staff meetings at the hospital. They were "on service" several months a year. During this time they had to see "service patients" (people who could not pay for medical care) both in the clinic and on the ward, without charge. When their patients were discharged they had to write lengthy summaries detailing the reasons for hospitalization, the treatment given and the condition at discharge. These rules were strictly enforced by the Joint Commission for the Accreditation of Hospitals, which periodically examined a hospital's records. Failure to comply meant loss of a hospital's national accreditation.

Doctors were busy people who hated to spend the time on all the necessary paperwork. Many had huge numbers of incomplete charts piling up in the record room. It was the responsibility of the chiefs to see that the doctors in their department completed their charts and lived up to their other responsibilities. Chiefs had the power to suspend the privileges of any doctor who did not do so, which meant that he/she could not admit patients to the hospital. We also were responsible for standards of care on our service. We had the power to prevent a doctor from carrying out any treatment that was considered dangerous or inappropriate. This of course could be appealed and was subject to review by the executive committees of the departments and of the hospital.

We chaired the monthly business meeting and arranged for speakers and topics for the weekly Grand Rounds, a clinical meeting where problem cases or interesting diagnoses or advances in medicine were discussed. We had to attend innumerable committee meetings, executive meetings, patient care review meetings, reviews of morbidity and mortality. We were supposed to take action on any problem that was identified in our department. It took up an enormous amount of time, for which we were not paid. Many chiefs coped by ignoring all but the most pressing problems since the time spent was time away from their practices. I found the work exhausting and had less time to spend at home with my family. I had to rearrange my office hours to fit my new responsibilities.

Al had been elected chief of Internal Medicine about a year before I became chief of Pediatrics. The controversy in his department was even more heated than in mine. Everyone recognized that Al in his quiet way could be fair to both sides in the debates about the expansion of the hospital and the proposed affiliation with a medical school. He had served on various committees and had been active in improving standards of care. A residency in Internal Medicine was already in existence and the residents considered Al one of their best teachers. His method of practice and of teaching was unusual in many ways. Al was the only doctor I know who continued to make house calls every day, literally to the last day of his life. He always felt that his elderly patients should not have the added stress of going to a doctor's office when they were ill. He emphasized to the residents that the interests of the patients were paramount, and he practiced what he preached, often to the detriment of his family. But his patients truly loved him and were incredibly loyal. Westfield has many executives who commute to New York. I know of several instances where an individual refused a promotion because it meant moving to a different area, and their family felt they could never find another doctor like Al.

When he was nominated to be chief, he was elected unanimously. I greatly regretted that Al was so modest and had no interest in seeking honors. He had made some very astute and unusual diagnoses which had saved the lives of many people. Because of this and his general abilities, one of the senior physicians wanted to propose him for membership in the American College of Physicians, an honor society which included the best physicians in the country. Al wouldn't even fill out the application.

With these new responsibilities, Al also had to rearrange his office hours. Seeing patients, caring for his mother, and hospital duties kept him busy from early morning until late night. I became increasingly grateful for his observance of the Sabbath, the one day that the family had time to be together. During the week Al and I were more likely to see one another at the hospital than at home with the children.

The chiefs of all the departments were asked to review the blueprints for the expansion of the hospital. Al and I noticed that the medical library, a small hole-in-the-wall next to the doctor's lounge, was unchanged while the lounge had been expanded to three times its size. We went on a vigorous campaign for a decent library. "But we don't have any more space," was the reply. We took a copy of the blueprints home and reconfigured the plan, enlarging the library at the expense of the lounge. We submitted it with our opinion that no medical college would be interested in affiliating with a hospital that didn't have an adequate library. Our plan was adopted. The delighted librarian said the library should be named for us.

I was troubled by the inadequate lighting over the children's beds and in the examining and treatment rooms on the pediatric ward. The pediatrics staff had been complaining and sending resolutions to the administration for some time but nothing had been done. Other areas of the hospital such as surgery received immediate attention when such complaints were made. I did not begrudge them this but felt that pediatrics was habitually ignored.

I knew that very specific requirements for physical facilities such as the space between beds, the square feet necessary for a nursery, etc., were part of the codes written by the Joint Commission and/or the Academy of Pediatrics. I checked the code books and found a lengthy section devoted to lighting requirements, spelled out in lumens. At my request the engineering department of the hospital gave me a written report of the lighting that existed on the pediatric floor. It was grossly inadequate. I sent a copy of the report to the administration with a copy of the requirements, and a memorandum that was a thinly-veiled threat that this inadequacy would be brought to the attention of the Joint Commission at their next visit.

A few days later I was asked to come to the office of the CEO, Bob Heinlein. Although I knew him from the many meetings we attended, I had never been in his office, and had never spoken to him. I was frightened. Perhaps my threat of whistle-blowing had carried things too far. He was standing with his hands clasped behind his back, a tall, formidable, authoritarian figure. He was still a relatively young man, probably in his early fifties, with only a hint of gray at the temples, where his brown hair was getting a bit thin. His face rarely gave any hint of what he was thinking. I couldn't tell whether or not he was angry. He courteously introduced the medical director, a physician I also knew only by sight, who was seated in one of the red leather armchairs in Heinlein's large, elegantly-furnished office. We all sat down on chairs drawn together to form a cozy little circle. The medical director did all the talking. It did not concern the lighting problem at all.

"Gloria," he said, "we've gotten a wonderful offer from Company X (one of the largest makers of infant formula.) They are going to supply all our formula needs without charge and send each mother home with a week's supply if we use only their brand in our nursery. We want you to see that this is approved at the next pediatrics business meeting."

"No," I said, "I think it's a bad idea. It will discourage women from breast feeding and if a doctor wants to order formula he wants the right to pick the formula of his choice. The company knows that if an infant is started on a specific formula and sent home with a free supply, the mother will probably continue using that brand for the rest of the first year."

Both men looked at me with astonishment. The chiefs had a reputation for carrying out the wishes of the administration. To have a brand new chief—and the first woman to have that role—refuse their initial request was unexpected. The medical director smiled at me ingratiatingly. "Do you realize how much money this would save for the hospital? Why, it would probably pay the cost of installing new lighting on the pediatric floor!"

I became angry. "Adequate lighting is the hospital's responsibility. It has nothing to do with saving money on formula! The way you try to cut costs on pediatrics is disgraceful!"

The medical director said, "Well, if you won't propose the idea, would you mind if I come to the next business meeting and propose it?"

"Be my guest," I said. "The meeting is this Friday. I'll put you on the agenda."

When we got up to leave, Heinlein said nothing except the customary goodbyes, but I thought I detected a glint of amusement in his eyes.

I wrote up the agenda without specifying why the Medical Director wanted to speak to the department. I introduced him without comment. As he began to outline his proposal, there were mutterings of unrest among the pediatricians. He never got to finish. The outburst of fury was spontaneous. It was difficult to restore order. Half-laughing, half-serious, he said, "Gloria, get me out of here before they lynch me!"

Al, greatly respected at the hospital, was always very formal with most of his colleagues and his patients. Few people realized he had an outrageous sense of humor which could manifest itself at the most unexpected times. This was less likely to happen at the hospital, but at the synagogue one Sabbath morning Rabbi Zell during his sermon, made some analogy to the benefits of chicken soup. "It has been shown to have great medicinal value, isn't that so, Dr. Schrager?"

Al slowly rose to his full 6'4" height, folding his arms and nodding gravely. "Yes," he said, "in fact we're presently trying to develop an intravenous form of chicken soup. But we've run into difficulty. We can't find a way of getting the noodles through the needle." There was a moment of stunned silence followed by an outburst of laughter from the entire congregation.

Internal Medicine was the first department to have a full-time director. Dr William (Bill) Minogue, an internist from Westfield, had decided to leave private practice and direct Overlook's transition to a teaching hospital. He served in the double capacity of head of the Department of Internal Medicine and director of medical education. His goal was to get full-time salaried directors for all the major disciplines, and he encouraged me to request one for pediatrics. Our department was not high on the administration's list of priorities. Pediatrics was a step-child in the allotment of funds since medicine and surgery brought in much more money. I broached the idea of a salaried director to the pediatrics attending staff and they were receptive, but pessimistic. At the monthly business meeting they decided that perhaps the administration would approve a part-time director. "Why don't we ask for half-time and be ready to settle for someone who could be here quarter-time."

I agreed and requested a hearing before the next meeting of the Board of Trustees. This was my first appearance before the Board, a group of influential men from the surrounding area, several of them CEOs of the large pharmaceutical companies that had their headquarters in New Jersey. The president of the Board was Bob Mulreany, a lawyer who lived in

Westfield. He was chief counsel for Columbia University. I was quite nervous and gave my little speech in a quavering voice. Mulreany jumped on me as if I were a hostile witness in a court room. "Out of the question," he barked. "Pediatrics does not make money for the hospital and we have other priorities."

I felt my temper rising, but knew I had to control it. "You've just spent over a million dollars on a new lobby and auditorium," I said coolly. "They don't bring in any money either. If you're trying to impress the community, I think they would be more impressed by good medical care for their children."

There was dead silence. Then Mulreany spoke. "Well, we'll consider it. You want a half-time director, right?"

"No," I answered, "We need a full-time director: half-time isn't good enough."

We were approved for full-time. Mulreany became one of my biggest supporters. A search committee was formed to interview candidates for the position of director of pediatrics and I was supposed to chair it. Bill Minogue came into my office and said he wanted me to resign from the committee. I was astonished.

"Why should I do that?" I asked.

He answered: "Because I want you to apply for the position yourself."

Al and I discussed the idea. He was not at all enthusiastic. We enjoyed practicing side by side, often sharing in the medical care of families. It was a pleasant arrangement. I would be downstairs in the office when our children came home from school and I would take some time off to go upstairs, hand out the milk and cookies and hear the events of the day. As full-time director, I would have even less time to spend with Al and the children. Fortunately the boys were now teenagers and were asserting their independence.

It was difficult to reach a decision. I enjoyed private practice and was very fond of my patients. Many had become almost like extended family. Although I might miss them and the office camaraderie, conditions upstairs with our multiple elderly boarders made the idea of full-time employment elsewhere increasingly attractive. I decided to apply for the newly-created position of Director of Pediatrics.

CHAPTER ELEVEN

Director of Pediatrics

When Bill Minogue asked me to apply, I recognized that there were challenges implicit in this new position that attracted me greatly. After spending two years as chief I felt that I knew what the problems were and how to go about solving them. I had certain goals in mind for the department. As chief I had been an elected official in what was really a volunteer unpaid position. I had neither the time nor the authority to institute necessary changes. That was the difference between a chief and a director. The former was a doctor whose first priority was his/her private practice and whose time-consuming hospital duties were secondary. The latter was a full-time paid employee whose primary responsibility was the hospital and its patients and who could spend all her energies in getting things done.

Pediatrics had never had much influence in formulating hospital policies or budgets. I was determined to make it a force to be reckoned with. One of my first concerns was that adult specialists were looking after children. Pediatric subspecialties were just beginning to develop and were centered mostly in the universities. There was not enough demand for their services to justify a subspecialist setting up practice in the suburbs. These were certified pediatricians who had further training in various medical fields: children's heart disease, kidney disease, endocrine problems including diabetes, gastro-intestinal disturbances, blood diseases including leukemia and other forms of cancer, allergies including asthma and other lung diseases, genetics, and the rheumatic and infectious diseases related to children. In our area, children who needed a specialist's care were usually seen by doctors trained to treat adults, who thought of children as little adults.

As chief, I had stopped a urologist from operating on a newborn who hadn't urinated in the first twenty-four hours. He simply considered the baby to have the same urological problems that afflict adults. This gentleman fit the Hollywood perception of a society doctor. Black hair slicked back, a flower in the buttonhole of his impeccably tailored suit, he had his own retinue of adoring nurses who followed him with memo pads to take down his orders and instructions. He called them all (as well as every other female on the staff) "dearie" or "sweetheart." To show his affection he would occasionally slap one of them on the rear.

The morning of our little contretemps, I was making my customary early rounds in the nursery and was just in time to see an infant being wheeled out in his crib.

"Where is he going?" I asked.

"To the OR. He hasn't voided in twenty-four hours and they want to dilate his urethra. The mother has signed consent."

"Take him back to the nursery. We have to discuss this further."

I began making phone calls to the baby's pediatrician and to the chief of surgery. (Urology was a subsection of the department of surgery, and their chief was responsible for standards of care in his department just as I was in pediatrics.)

The door to the nursery suddenly burst open, admitting the livid urologist in his OR scrub suit.

"How dare you interfere with my operating schedule? You have no authority to do that! Have you gone crazy? I'm calling the medical director immediately!"

"Go right ahead," I said calmly. "I've already called the chief of surgery and the baby's pediatrician. We'll all have a nice little talk before you touch this baby."

A short time later we were all gathered around the baby's crib in heated discussion. I was trying to explain that occasionally during the birth process an infant might urinate without anyone noticing it and it might be a while before another urination was recorded. We were so absorbed in argument we had forgotten to diaper the baby after examining him. Suddenly he let forth a mighty stream that with unerring aim caught the urologist full in the face, to my intense satisfaction.

Of course, not all problems could be solved this easily. Although we had not yet achieved a medical school affiliation, I had many contacts at both UMDNJ (The University of Medicine and Dentistry of New Jersey) and Columbia, and I was anxious to arrange for pediatrics subspecialists to have consulting privileges at Overlook. Many of the adult specialists resisted the idea. It did not contribute to my popularity and was the source of much friction.

Despite their resistance, I stubbornly persisted. Pediatrics subspecialists were necessary to institute a recognized teaching program in pediatrics. Such a program would improve the quality of care of hospitalized children. It required the presence of residents trained in an accredited hospital residency, who would be available to care for children twenty-four hours a day. Doctors saw their hospitalized patients for only a short time each day before hurrying back to their offices. To have trained doctors present at all times to check on patients and treat emergencies was highly desirable.

It was not only necessary to train residents but it was also important to institute a program of continuing medical education for the attending staff of physicians. Progress in medicine was dramatic and it was difficult for practicing physicians to keep up with the latest advances. Many procedures they learned during their training were now considered obsolete or unnecessary. Examples were routine tonsillectomies, the repair of umbilical hernias (protrusions from the navel) and a host of urological procedures for incontinence and urinary tract infections.

It would be simplistic to say that doctors continued doing these unnecessary procedures for financial gain. This may have been true for a small number of physicians, but most were decent, honorable men and women who would not subject a patient to the risks and discomforts of a procedure they considered unnecessary. They had learned that these procedures were important when they were in training and they had continued doing them.

As chief, and even as director, I did not have the power to interfere with the way doctors treated their private patients unless an acute threat existed. But as director I scheduled the weekly Ground Rounds that were a requirement of the department. Some of these meetings could be devoted to a discussion of these issues.

There were still times when these controversial procedures were necessary. But the reasons for doing them were limited. A meeting that discussed this made it more difficult for a doctor to justify a procedure that was not in accordance with the general consensus.

It was relatively easy to organize conferences and invite guest speakers whose prestige could influence the way we practiced. It was much more difficult to work for the accreditation of a pediatric residency and a university affiliation. When I had submitted my application for the position of director, I knew that there were several male applicants who were being considered more favorably. I have no illusions as to why I was chosen. The salary offered was much less than one could make in private practice. Job security depended on being successful in developing an accredited residency program and none of the other candidates thought this could be accomplished. In short, I was chosen by default.

I had been in private practice for almost 20 years—from 1953 to 1972. Some of the children I had cared for were now grown and married and had their own children, many of whom had become my patients. I sent everyone a letter of farewell, explaining that I would be at Overlook full-time and could no longer continue a private practice. Many wrote me fond letters in response. The ones I treasured the most were the painstakingly printed, badly misspelled letters of the children.

Leaving was made somewhat easier because I knew my patients would be in good hands. I gave all my records to Dr. Carolkay Lissenden, a good friend, whose method of practice and relationship with her patients were similar to mine. Carolkay said she would keep these records separate from hers for several years "just in case things don't work out and you want to come back." My guilt at abandoning Al in our private practice was quickly assuaged. When I finally did get the job, he promptly took over my office and all other available space, happy with his expanded quarters and the unaccustomed quiet—no more pediatric patients.

One of my first experiences as full-time director was to attend a hospital weekend retreat at a think tank in Sterling Forest, a couple of hours north of us. It was a meeting to discuss hospital policy and plans for the future and included administration executives, members of the Board of Trustees, and the chiefs and/or directors of the various departments. We were all colleagues and we got along well, but it was obvious that they regarded me first as a woman and only secondarily as a doctor.

I was the only woman present. It was apparent immediately that the director of the think tank was not pleased by this invasion of his bachelor quarters. He opened the meeting with a long introductory speech, liberally peppered with locker room obscenities. I remained relaxed and cool but noted that the other participants were avoiding my gaze. When we broke for refreshments, several came over to me to apologize for his behavior. "Forget it," I said. "He hasn't said anything I haven't heard before."

Many considered this man the hospital's guru, but I was not impressed. I thought his actions were bizarre. He said he used the vernacular to put everyone at ease but I didn't think that was the case. He made me feel decidedly unwelcome and embarrassed the others.

I had to attend frequent dinner meetings at which I was the only woman present. Several hospitals were represented at one of these meetings. We had met to exchange views about problems in our area and I was seated next to the director of a neighboring institution. He started to lecture me on the reasons why medical schools should not admit women. I had heard this many times before and considered argument unprofitable since neither of us would be influenced by the other.

I attempted another subject, but my dinner companion returned to the theme with variations. His voice became louder and louder under the influence, I suspect, of the prolonged cocktail hour that had preceded dinner. He said, "You women think you're the equal of men but you're not. You never were and you never will be."

I turned away, saying, "Enough. I only discuss these matters with my equals."

Purple with fury, he half-rose from his chair, bellowing," Are you saying I'm not your equal?"

I did not enjoy these events and avoided them when I could.

"No," I said, "you're saying it."

The meeting I resented most, ever since we joined the Overlook staff in 1953, was the annual dinner meeting. It was held at a country club whose membership was restricted,

WESTFIELD LEADER, 1972

Focus on Medical Education

With the appointment of Dr. Gloria Schrager, well known Westfield pediatrician, to the new post of Pediatric Director of Education, Overlook Hospital moves to an important new level both in quality patient care and in its medical education programming.

Dr. Schrager has challenging ideas for Overlook's pediatric department. "There have been tremendous advances in medicine today, but many have not yet been applied to pediatrics at the suburban hospital level," she points out. "New concepts have brought a dramatic decrease in neonatal mortality. This is one of the main areas where I hope to concentrate," Dr. Schrager emphasized, explaining new techniques of constant monitoring of high risk new-borns to maintain blood oxygen levels, temperature, respiration, heart rate, acid-base balance and other complexities, requiring constant professional supervision.

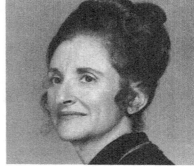

Gloria O. Schrager, M.D. Director of Pediatrics

"The opposite end of the pediatric spectrum also needs attention, the field of adolescent medicine — perhaps a clinic where kids can just come in with their problems — acne, drugs, sex, whatever," she explained; also a separated area for in-hospital adolescent patients.

A Child Evaluation Clinic for children with learning disabilities is another main goal which has been under study. Here, the combined skills of the pediatrician, neurologist, and psychiatrist will seek to determine how much of the child's problem is functional, metabolic or emotional and apply the team approach to teach children to function at their best possible capacity.

Dr. Schrager's assignment will relate directly to Overlook's increasing ties with the New Jersey College of Medicine. The hospital is currently applying for A.M.A. approved residencies in pediatrics in order to provide a flow of incoming pediatricians.

A native New Yorker, brought up in the Adirondacks, Dr. Schrager earned her medical degree at Woman's Medical College in Philadelphia. She met her husband Alvin Schrager, M.D., former Chief of the Dept. of Internal Medicine at Overlook, while interning at Metropolitan Hospital in New York City, where she also took her residency in pediatrics, followed by a fellowship at New York Hospital-Cornell Medical School.

Mother of two sons, Ralph and Lewis, respectively a sophomore and senior at Westfield High, Dr. Schrager is an ardent outdoorswoman and swimming-camping-skiing enthusiast.

although the Jewish, Italian and the two African-American doctors on the staff were graciously welcomed for the evening as guests. Wives were not invited. Dress was strictly formal. Al hated to go, but a lot of networking went on at the meeting and, as new members of the staff, I thought it important that we attend. Besides, I wanted them to know that their good ol' boys' club now included a woman who knew how to dress in a formal evening gown. When I became Director of Pediatrics, one of my little extra projects was to change the location of the meeting and to have women invited. It took several years and I ran into fierce opposition, but when it was finally accomplished, several of the most resistant members of the staff reluctantly admitted that now the evening was much more enjoyable.

I found that I had an easier time at the necessary dinner meetings if I dressed attractively. This held true also for appearances before various policy-making or influential groups like the Board of Trustees. Sometimes it seemed that I was spending more time on my wardrobe and how I did my hair than on the presentation I had to make. It amused Al greatly. When I began to worry over the outcome of some meeting he would laugh and say, "Just wear your pink suit." I had a pink ultrasuede suit that I wore with a lace blouse and a cameo pin. The outfit went well with my long dark hair that I wore in a French knot or a braid in back. The stratagem seemed to work. If I had to succeed in a sexist society, two could play at that game.

We knew that our chances of getting residents would be greater if we had an affiliation with a medical school. We made a proposal to the University of Medicine and Dentistry in New Jersey. Contract discussions dragged on interminably. One afternoon, after an unproductive meeting, we received an ultimatum: the medical school would have complete control over our hospital—"take it or leave it." Bill Minogue, an Irishman not to be trifled with, turned heel without a word and left followed by the rest of Overlook's contingent.

We were frustrated and discouraged, but Bob Mulreany, general counsel for Columbia University and head of our Board of Trustees, stepped into the breach. At a meeting to discuss alternatives to our affiliation with UMDNJ, he suddenly proposed,

OVERLOOK STAFF DINNER 1972

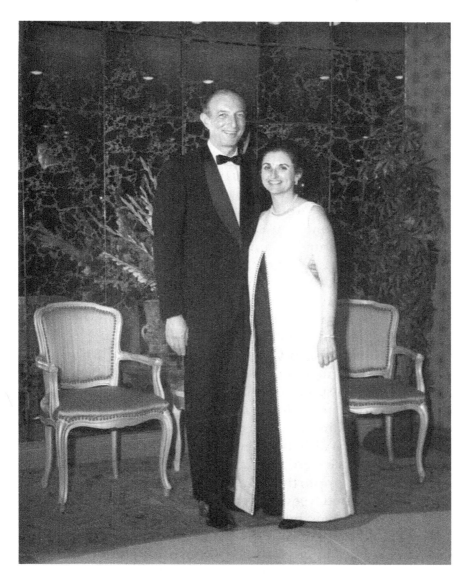

"Why don't we affiliate with Columbia?" Many of us had ties with Columbia but an official affiliation with that prestigious institution did not seem possible. We happened to be in the right place at the right time. The importance of primary care (the care of the whole patient, by doctors who did not specialize) was being recognized at last and the government was granting large sums to medical schools who would provide this training to their students. Columbia had always been a tertiary care center, the students trained by doctors doing research or sub-specializing. Students there had minimal exposure to internists and pediatricians in routine office practice.

Columbia was anxious to remedy this situation and be eligible for primary care grants. Affiliation with a community hospital fit their needs as much as their expertise fit ours. Contract discussions were brief and amicable, helped of course by Bob Mulreany. In 1975, we became Columbia's first community affiliate. Students and house staff began taking elective rotations at Overlook although it meant making the long trek from Manhattan. They spent time in the hospital and in the offices of private doctors and sent back enthusiastic reports. We were a popular elective and the directors of the departments involved were given faculty rank. I became an associate professor. Several years later, I was promoted to full professor.

Our affiliation with Columbia was everything I hoped for. Dr. Richard Behrman, Professor and Chairman of Pediatrics at the time, was very supportive and gave me invaluable advice about getting accreditation for a residency in pediatrics. He also encouraged Columbia medical students and residents to take elective rotations with us, and was pleased that their evaluations of the experience were very favorable. Other faculty members were equally supportive. Dr. Welton Gersony, Director of Cardiology, visited frequently, not only to conduct conferences and do consultations, but to chair a monthly meeting on medical ethics. Drs. Marty Nash and Bob Seigle, pediatrics nephrologists, held weekly teaching conferences for the residents and saw patients in consultation. All became good friends, and when I went to Columbia to attend meetings, I felt as much at home as I did at Overlook.

WESTFIELD LEADER, 1984

Dr. Schrager Promoted To Full Professor

Gloria O. Schrager M.D. of Westfield, director of pediatrics at Overlook Hospital, has been promoted to clinical professor of pediatrics at Columbia University College of Physicians and Surgeons.

Dr. Schrager was in private practice and served as the elected chief of the pediatric department at Overlook unitl 1972 when she was chosen to become the full-time director of pediatrics. She was named an associate clinical professor at the time of Overlook's major major teaching affiliation with Columbia in 1974, and held that rank until her present promotion.

Dr. Schrager is one of four physicians at Overlook to achieve full professional status at Columbis — Michael Bernstein, M.D., chairman of the department of medical education; William F. Minogue, M.D., vice president of medical affairs; and Richard W. Brenner, M.D., director of surgical education, also hold that rank.

As director of pediatrics, Dr. Schrager is responsible for standards of pediatric care at Overlook Hospital. She is program chairman of the fully accredited pediatric residency training program at Overlook and is also responsible for the pediatric instruction of residents in family practice and emergency medicine. In addition, Columbia University medical students come to Overlook for her program in pediatric physical diagnosis and for experience in community pediatrics.

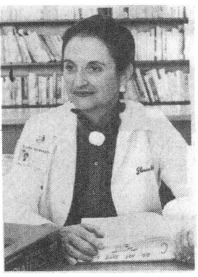

Dr.Gloria O. Schrager

Dr. Schrager's promotion also includes full attending physician status at the Babies Hospital of Columbia Presbyterian Medical Center in New York City.

143

CHAPTER TWELVE

The Pediatric Residency

I considered accreditation for a pediatric residency vital in achieving my goal of a reputable teaching service. I filled out the voluminous applications and was rejected. Most pediatric residencies were situated in university teaching centers. An independent residency in pediatrics at a community hospital was practically unheard-of. The Accreditation Counsel for Graduate Medical Education (ACGME) considered us ineligible for a variety of reasons. They listed as deficiencies the lack of adequate volume of patients, the lack of exposure to a wide variety of cases for resident experience, and the lack of pediatric subspecialists. They were also concerned by the apparent inadequate experience in ambulatory care in well-baby clinics, in the emergency room and in subspecialty clinics. I appealed, submitting data to show that with our Columbia affiliation and other changes I had inaugurated, those deficiencies had been corrected.

The ACGME asked us to appear before a special appeals panel at AMA headquarters in Chicago. Bill Minogue, Bob Heinlein and I flew to Chicago and registered at the entrance.

"Oh yes, doctors, you're expected, go right up," said the security officer. Turning to me he said, "And you, miss, can wait in the visitors' waiting room." Heinlein and Minogue hastily corrected this misapprehension, but when we got upstairs, the chairman of the appeals panel shook hands cordially with them, ignoring me. Again, explanations had to be made.

The application was rejected multiple times. It got to the point where I was commuting frequently to Chicago, catching a 6 AM flight out of Newark to be in Chicago when the offices opened and coming home exhausted the same evening. I think they finally agreed to accept the residency on probation because they were tired of my constant reappearances and were sure that on detailed inspection two years later at the end of the probationary period, it would be found deficient.

With this provisional acceptance I was able to hire residents. I set about strengthening the program, arranging for the residents to rotate through Columbia for certain subspecialties. Columbia pediatric subspecialists also came out to Overlook to teach and consult in subspecialty clinics. The ambulatory experience of the residents was strengthened not only by these clinics but by the increased presence of the pediatrics residents in the emergency room.

Emergency rooms in those days were not organized to treat children. ER doctors had no pediatrics training and most of them treated children like little adults—and very uncooperative, annoying little adults at that. The emergency room experience for children could be disastrous. They were often placed next to critically ill adults and the urgent, emotional scenes around them increased their fright and confusion. The standard equipment in the ER did not include children's sizes and although bones could be set and lacerations stitched with the equipment on hand, other equipment for intravenous therapy, CPR, and a host of other emergencies was not available.

After some difficulties I was able to convince the director of the Emergency Room to set aside a special space for children, somewhat apart from the general hubbub. We decorated it with colorful children's murals. I worked with the ER staff to create a "pediatrics crash cart," a moveable equipment cart that contained pediatric doses of emergency drugs and children's sizes of emergency equipment. In addition, I arranged for a senior pediatric resident to be called for all pediatric emergencies. This benefited all concerned. The residents gained more experience and training, the emergency room doctors had their patient responsibilities decreased, and the children had a less frightening experience.

Shortly after we had established this cooperatve effort with the emergency department, we had our first real test of the system. A two-year-old boy was admitted in shock. He had been involved in a bizarre auto accident. His mother had driven to the home of a child who was in their carpool and had parked in the driveway. She left her little boy unattended on the front seat of the car for just a moment, to pick up the other child. These were the days before we had car seats for children and the little boy had promptly climbed into the driver's seat and released the brake. The driveway was on a steep hill, causing the car to begin a slow roll down to the street. The horrified mother, nine months pregnant, ran back to the car, opened the door, and yanked the child out, falling heavily on top of him. When they arrived in the Emergency Department, the child was unconscious and had signs of internal bleeding. We started immediate treatment for shock, using our brand new pediatrics crash cart, and were able to stabilize his blood pressure in the emergency room. We typed and cross-matched him for a blood transfusion and then rushed him directly to the OR where a team of doctors and nurses were waiting. They found multiple areas of bleeding involving several torn blood vessels and lacerations of the right lobe of the liver. But when these were repaired, bleeding did not stop, shock continued, and more blood had to be given. Further investigation revealed that the dome of the liver had been fractured. The boy's chest had to be opened and a third of the right lobe of his liver removed through the chest incision. It was the only way it could be reached. Several loops of intestine were also badly torn and had to be cut away, and the remaining intestines reconnected. His post-operative course was very stormy with many complications. We all recognized that his chances for survival were slim. He had many metabolic problems, severe infections, and could not be fed by mouth. Several members of the hospital staff—surgeons, nurses and residents—were at his bedside continuously. He gradually improved and was finally discharged in good condition on the 80th hospital day. He insisted on toddling out of the hospital "by myself," although he agreed to hold his parents' hands. Under no conditions would he allow himself to be carried.

The most dramatic change in the pediatric department was in the growth of the subspecialty clinics. The Columbia faculty, from Dr. Richard Behrman, the chairman, to most of subspecialists, were very supportive and visited frequently. Many became good friends. The pediatricians at Overlook were delighted that they no longer had to send their patients to New York for consultations, and families were pleased that they could get that degree of expertise locally.

I also arranged for the residents to serve as "junior partners" in the offices of a select group of attending pediatricians who were interested in teaching. These pediatricians received faculty rank at Columbia. The residents had weekly office hours with their preceptors and were able to follow their patients more closely than in the usual out-patient department of a large university hospital.

Two years later our application for full approval of the residency looked quite impressive. An inspector from the Residency Review Commission (RRC) came to Overlook, went over the data minutely, and then asked to meet with the residents in closed session. "This is where I get the real lowdown," he said. About two hours later he came to my office. "I usually come out of a resident session with a list of complaints about the weaknesses of the program. These residents, especially a very articulate, enthusiastic young man named John Vigorita, keep insisting that the program is even better than you say. I don't know whether they are all lying in their teeth but I have the distinct impression they would kill for you." We received full accreditation.

RESIDENTS' ROUNDS, OVERLOOK HOSPITAL, 1972

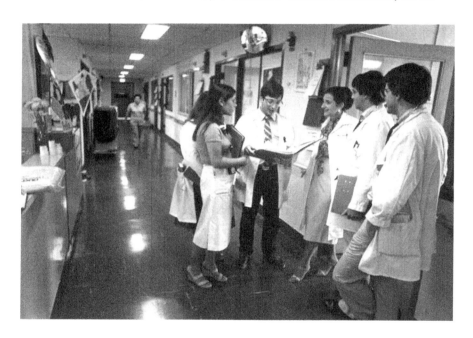

CHAPTER THIRTEEN

Financing the program

M y greatest concern was finding the funds to finance the various programs on my agenda. Pediatrics still did not have a high priority in the hospital's budget. My fund-raising efforts sought many sources. We received a $50,000 grant from the state to improve the nurseries. The Helena Rubenstein Foundation gave us funds for a fetal monitor. Parents of a teenager killed in a bicycle accident donated money for an adolescent unit, to be named in her memory. Grateful parents also helped us acquire sophisticated electroencephalographic equipment and other technology for intensive care of older children. The American Stock Exchange, chaired by Arthur Levitt, gave a large donation to our newly created Hematology/Oncology Center for children.

One of the most dramatic advances in pediatrics was the development of neonatology as a specialty. New methods and new technology were being used to treat infants at high risk because of prematurity, infection, birth trauma, etc. There were no neonatal intensive care units in community hospitals. We were supposed to transfer distressed newborns to large centers for care. But transfers took time and irreparable damage could occur if infants were not resuscitated and treated immediately, or at least had their conditions stabilized before transfer. I requested funds to have a neonatologist train the entire staff in the latest techniques and also to buy an infant respirator. The request was denied.

There were many volunteer organizations in the community. One was the Junior Fortnightly Club. Their members were collecting Betty Crocker food coupons which were redeemed by that company to finance any worthy community endeavor. I met

GLORIA O. SCHRAGER, M.D.

STARTING A NEONATAL INTENSIVE CARE UNIT WITH BETTY CROCKER FOOD STAMPS 1971

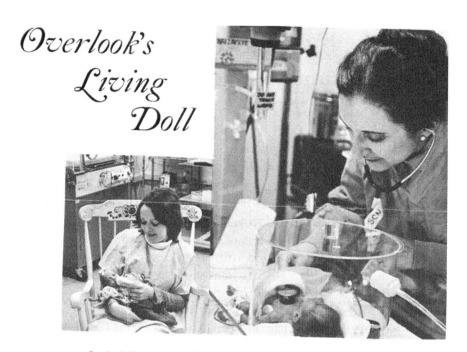

Overlook's Living Doll

Overlook Hospital has a living doll . . . Born three months premature, tiny Julia Elizabeth Artiglere weighed in at 2 lbs. on November 15. Julia recently passed the 4½ pound mark which meant graduation from Overlook's Neonatal Nursery where she has been a star boarder for two and a half months.

Dressed in doll's clothes purchased by her mother, the diminutive princess of the Overlook Nursery returned home to Lake Hopatcong with her overjoyed parents, Mr. and Mrs. Joseph Artiglere.

According to Dr. Gloria O. Schrager, Director of Pediatric Education at Overlook, Julia maintained life through the critical early period thanks to the Bourne Infant Respirator given to Overlook by the Junior Fortnightly Club of Summit, which is still raising funds for the respirator through the collection of Betty Crocker food stamps (stamps are welcome at the Fortnightly Club of Summit, or can be left at the Overlook Volunteer Office.)

"Respiration is perhaps the most critical problem for preemies," Dr. Schrager pointed out. "When necessary the artificial respirator can completely take over the breathing chores of an infant's immature lungs."

Julia is one of the smallest babies to pull through the trying ordeal of high risk prematurity in the unit's history.

Within four days of birth, Julia went down to a scant pound and a half. On November 19 she went on the critical list when she suffered difficulty in breathing. With a one in ten chance of survival, Julia fought back, constant focus of attention of a team of doctors and nurses who monitored her every breath for over ten weeks.

with the Club and asked them to use the coupons to pay for an infant respirator. They were excited by the project but apprehensive about their ability to collect enough stamps.

"How much does it cost?"

When I told them, they shook their heads.

"We could never collect that kind of money."

"Supposing I could convince the Administration to let you pay it off on the installment plan. Even if it takes several years, the respirator will still be saving babies' lives for a long time after you're finished."

They agreed to make the commitment if I could get the hospital to accept the idea. It was easier than I thought—probably because several women in the club were related to members of the Board of Trustees. People find it difficult to believe that the first respirator in Overlook's now highly sophisticated neonatal intensive care unit was paid for by Betty Crocker food coupons.

I received considerable criticism for daring to keep distressed newborns at Overlook instead of transferring them to large centers. I countered by showing them our statistics for neonatal mortality and morbidity which were on a par with the centers and much lower than most of the other community hospitals. And the parents were much happier being able to visit their babies close to home. We received some favorable publicity when a premature infant weighing less than two pounds was successfully resuscitated and survived, "a living doll" according to newspaper reports. Her mother went to the toy store to find a ruffled little doll's dress, to have her picture taken for the papers. Today such survival is not unusual. Back then it was considered little short of miraculous.

Probably my greatest challenge was convincing the Valerie Fund to inaugurate their service at Overlook. We had already created a subspecialty clinic for the diagnosis and treatment of children with cancer and blood disorders. It was run jointly by a part-time pediatric oncologist, Dr. George Gill, who was doing research at one of the pharmaceutical companies, and by specialists directed by Dr. James Wolff, Director of Pediatric Hematology/Oncology at Columbia.

The Valerie Fund had been formed to honor the memory of Valerie Goldstein, who had died after a long and gallant struggle with cancer. Her friends and family, influential members of the community, wanted to establish a center in New Jersey so that children with cancer would not have to make the long, difficult, sometimes daily trips to New York for treatment as Valerie had done. Members of their search committee had just about decided to start their center at another hospital but had been convinced to meet with Overlook personnel to see what we had to offer.

After a long exhausting meeting, I saw that their minds were still set on the other hospital. I began to lose patience and stopped pleading for their support. "Look," I said. "You can go to whatever hospital you choose and start a center from scratch. We have one already and we are continuing to expand it, so there will be two centers in the same area. That won't be good for either of them. If you come here we can build an outstanding program with our Columbia affiliation." They held some more meetings and decided to support us.

The Valerie Center grew at an astonishing rate and soon had its own staff of nurses and social workers. It was clear that we needed a full-time director, but Dr. Gill could not leave his research at the pharmaceutical company. I asked for advice from Jim Wolff, who had become a good friend at Columbia. He looked at me reflectively. "You know, Gloria," he said, "I'll soon be sixty-five and will have to step down as head of the department, although I can continue my research."

I was incredulous. "Jim," I said, "would you seriously consider becoming the full-time director of the Valerie Center?"

"Why don't you make me an offer?" he said. For once, there was no hesitation with the appropriation of funds, and Dr. Wolff left Columbia to direct the hematology-oncology program at Overlook.

The Center was adopted by the New York Giants football team, in 1977. These great burly men would come to the hospital to see the children, holding them with incredible gentleness. Each year they would hold a Roast at which some sports figure would be the target. As a benefit for our Center, these events became enormously popular and celebrities from different sports and the entertainment world attended. When my picture appeared in the paper, arm in arm with Phil Simms and Wilt Chamberlain, I think my children were more impressed than by anything else I had done.

VALERIE FUND ACTIVITIES

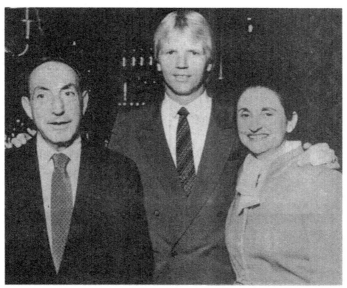

AT VALERIE FUND ROAST - Giants quarterback Phil Simms is flanked by Dr. James Wolff and Dr. Gloria Schrager during annual sports roast benefiting the Valerie Fund Center for Children's Cancer and Blood Disorders at Overlook Hospital. Dr. Wolff is Director of the Valerie Fund Center. Dr. Schrager is Director of Pediatrics at Overlook. This year's "roastee" was head coach Ray Perkins.

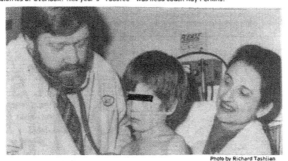

Photo by Richard Tashjian

Drs. George M. Gill and Gloria O. Schrager, both of whom are active in Overlook Hospital's child and adolescent cancer treatment program

A highly specialized child and adolescent cancer program, using the latest techniques in cancer treatment, has been created at Overlook Hospital in Summit.

Dr. Gloria O. Schrager, director of pediatric education, said the program is aimed at providing a regional center for children with malignant diseases, offering 24-hour care to an estimated caseload of more than 750 child and adolescent cancer patients in the state.

She also said the Overlook patients will have "the added backup and intensified skills" of the hospital's formal teaching affiliation with Columbia University's College of Physicians and Surgeons and Columbia Presbyterian Medical Center.

Dr. Donald F. Tapley, dean of the college, said the medical facility regards the affiliation "as a most significant advance in services available to child cancer patients in New Jersey."

"Overlook's affiliation with Colum-

bia will make our consultation services and treatment resources immediately available to Overlook physicians, their patients and their families," he declared.

Schrager stressed the new program will also employ a specially trained staff geared toward helping parents and children with emotional and psychological problems brought on by the impact of malignant diseases.

FULL-TIME DIRECTOR APPOINTED FOR CHILDREN CANCER CENTER
1981

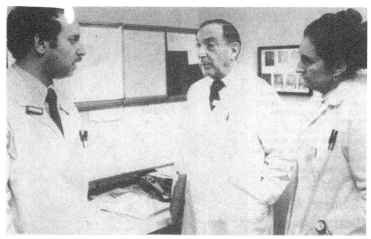

NEW DIRECTOR — Dr. James Wolff, center, director of the Valerie Children's Center for Cancer and Blood Disorders, consults with Dr. Louis Schwartz, pediatric radiotherapist, and Dr. Gloria Schrager, director of pediatrics at Overlook Hospital.

Full-Time Director Named At Overlook Valerie Clinic

James A. Wolff, M.D. professor of pediatrics at Columbia College of Physicians and Surgeons and a children's cancer specialist, has been named the full-time director of the Valerie Children's Center for Cancer and Blood Disorders at Overlook Hospital.

Dr. Wolff's appointment will result in the "dramatic expansion of services to Valerie Center patients," according to Gloria O. Schrager, M.D., director of pediatrics at Overlook. The Valerie Center was founded in 1977 as the Valerie Fund Children's Clinic to provide medical and psychological support services for young New Jersey cancer patients. Until the appointment of Dr. Wolff, it was operated on a limited basis with a part-time medical director.

The Valerie Center has been supported since its founding by the Valerie Fund, founded in memory of nine-year-old Valerie Goldstein of Watchung, who died of cancer before such a

treatment center existed in New Jersey. Members of the Fund are volunteers who raise money for the Center through a variety of events during the year, including a Sports Roast which attracts professional athletes, celebrities, political figures and thousands of guests each June.

Dr. Wolff will be joined at the Valerie Center by Fredrick Braun, M.D., a Board-certified pediatric hematologist/oncologist, and Louis Schwartz, M.D., one of a handful of pediatric radiotherapists in North America. The Valerie Center staff includes Emy Hyans, a pediatric social worker, and Kit Kenyon, a pediatric nurse practitioner.

Most Valerie Center patients recieve their treatment on an

outpatient basis after an initial brief period of hospitalization. Disruptions in their daily lives, including schooling, are kept to a minimum.

Dr. Wolff is the former director of the Division of Pediatric Hematology/Oncology at the Babies Hospital, Columbia Presbyterian Medical Center. He has been on the teaching staff at Columbia since 1949 and was a pioneer in the development of new treatments for children's cancer. He is a principal investigator for the national Children's Cancer Study Group, which makes recommendations on new treatment protocols.

Dr. Wolff is a graduate of Harvard University and the New York University College of Medicine.

In 1975, to increase community support and recognition of the hospital, I cooperated with the school system in Summit to organize a series of talks on the problems of adolescence. Sex education in the schools, birth control, drug addiction, and the rights of adolescents to confidentiality in medical care were the source of much anxiety and controversy among parents. The program was widely advertised and featured Overlook specialists in pediatrics, obstetrics and psychiatry. We included a lawyer from the Board of Trustees. The auditorium was packed to overflowing and many people had to be turned away. A drug company funded a booklet reprinting our speeches. The title of the book was *Coping With or Copping Out: Explorations in Human Understanding* and it was available without charge to all who attended the meeting. The response was overwhelming and we had to repeat the entire program in one of the school auditoriums several weeks later. The program was featured in many newspapers. They said it created a new tolerance and understanding of young people seeking medical advice and treatment without their parents' involvement. The reputation of the pediatric department at Overlook was growing.

CHAPTER FOURTEEN

Dr. Benjamin Spock

I had set specific goals for improving the pediatric service if I were appointed director. Among these goals was my aim to have our hospital and its pediatrics department recognized for its high standards of care. I wanted to carry out a program of continuing medical education that would be popular with pediatricians not only in New Jersey, but in neighboring states as well. I organized a widely publicized series of pediatric conferences to achieve this. Some of the most famous pediatricians in the country spoke at these meetings, including Dr. Sydney Gellis, editor of the Yearbook of Pediatrics, famous for his biting wit and encyclopedic knowledge.

In 1980, the most notable of these meetings featured Dr. Benjamin Spock. Dr. Spock was the author of *Baby and Child Care*, a book that had become the bible for young parents. It had sold over 28 million copies and been translated into 26 languages. He had recently published another book, *Raising Children in a Difficult Time*. His books were filled with common sense advice about the problems of parenting. He tried to instill a feeling of self-confidence in young parents. The opening sentence of *Baby and Child Care* had become a classic: "You know more than you think you do."

Dr. Spock was living in semi-retirement in Arkansas with his wife Mary and her teenage daughter. He agreed to spend several days with us, and I decided to take full advantage of his visit. I organized several seminars for physicians, an open meeting for the public at large, and hospital rounds where he could personally meet the residents, students and patients.

DR. SPOCK VISITS OVERLOOK
1980

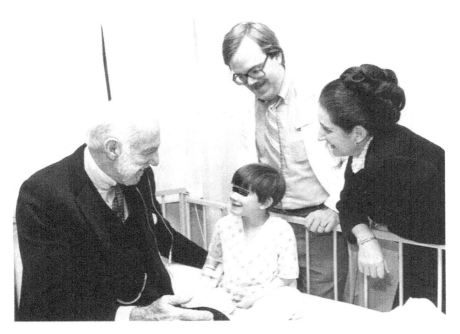

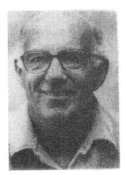

Dr. Benjamin Spock

Dr. Spock
to speak at
Overlook

AREA — Dr. Benjamin Spock, pediatrician and author, will headline an all-day seminar on pediatrics at Overlook Hospital on Wednesday, April 23.

The public is invited to attend an evening lecture by Dr. Spock, who will speak on "Child Rearing: Yesterday and Today," at 8 p.m., in Overlook's Wallace Auditorium.

"The program with Dr. Spock may help to dispel some of the misinterpretations of his theories on child rearing," said Gloria O. Schrager, M.D., director of pediatrics at Overlook. "Whether or not you agree with him, Dr. Spock has earned the reputation as being concerned with children and their welfare. And his book on child rearing helped free parents from some of the rigid rules they were taught-

The highlight was the large evening meeting to which the entire community was invited. The auditorium was packed and we jerry-rigged loudspeakers in the lobby for the overflow crowd. Spock was still a controversial figure and several members of the Board of Trustees objected to his presence. He had opposed the Vietnam War and had run for President in 1972 as the candidate of the Peace and Freedom Party. His campaign had attracted a lot of young people, some of them beatniks involved in the drug scene. Conservative America blamed him and his teachings for creating a climate of permissiveness that had affected a whole generation of rebellious youth.

Anyone who had read his books knew that this was untrue. Spock had always advocated establishing boundaries of acceptable behavior and had emphasized the importance of consistency in teaching children to observe them. He believed that children should respect their parents but that parents also had to respect the growing development of their children.

Although much of the heated controversy had died down, he was still a well-known personality, frequently referred to in the press, usually by people who had never read and failed to understand his teachings. Members of the community who objected to his speaking at Overlook were particularly unhappy with the theme I had chosen for his series of talks: *The Pediatrician as Child Advocate and Instrument for Social Change.*

They urged Bob Heinlein to stop the meetings. My admiration for Heinlein increased when he solidly supported me despite his conservative leanings. I don't think he really approved of Spock and his views (or what he thought he knew about them.) He certainly disapproved of Spock's role in the anti-war movement. But he believed directors should be given as much autonomy as possible in developing their programs and he would not interfere.

All the local newspapers carried large features about Spock. Many distorted his message and what he had always believed in. One carried a large headline, "Dr. Spock changes his tune—parents must be firm," he says. The article started out by saying, "The man credited with opening the floodgates of permissiveness in child rearing . . . now spends most of his time on the podium telling parents to be firm with their kids." In his interviews with reporters, Spock claimed he had been first labeled permissive by the Reverend Norman Vincent Peale, "a scalawag who poses as a divine."

Spock defended his philosophy on child care, which had remained consistent. However, he did apologize for the sexist tone of the earlier editions of his book. He said, "I wrote some foolishly sexist things before I was wised up by the women's movement around 1970." He said he had been attacked by Gloria Steinem who had labeled him "an oppressor of women in the same category as Sigmund Freud." He laughed and said he had been flattered by the comparison but he did revise his book in 1978, eliminating the sex-typing and the exclusive use of the male pronoun.

I had reserved rooms for Spock at a hotel near the hospital but when we spoke by phone before his visit, he said, "I'd much rather stay in your home, Gloria, if you'll have me." Al and I were delighted and hosted our famous guest for several days. Although we would be having lunch and dinner with various groups, I wanted to be sure he had a good breakfast before the day started and phoned his wife Mary to discuss his preferences. Mary told me he always had a special steel-ground oatmeal for breakfast.

Oatmeal was a staple in our house but this special variety was unknown to me, as it was to the multiple stores and supermarkets we tried. Finally Al had the brilliant idea of phoning a drug store that also stocked health foods.

"Sure we have it, doc," was the reply. "You can pick it up in the morning. I'm just locking up for the night." Al explained he needed it immediately since our guest, Dr. Spock, would be breakfasting with us early the next morning. "For Dr. Spock?" was the awed response. "For Dr. Spock I'll wait 'til you get here and you can have it gratis, with my compliments."

Al jokingly complained, for years after, that for his breakfast I would make the quick-cooking three-minute oatmeal, but for Dr. Spock I got up an hour earlier to slowly simmer his special steel-ground variety.

One of the TV talk shows, learning of Spock's presence in the metropolitan area, asked him to appear live in their New

York studios for an interview. I drove him into Manhattan, basking in reflected glory as we lunched and walked through the streets of Manhattan, his tall figure instantly recognizable. On the way home we were stuck in rush-hour traffic and we had a long time to talk. He told me something of his life and how he happened to write his books. In semi-retirement now, he told me about living in Arkansas with his second wife, Mary, and her teenage daughter. He had several grown sons from his first marriage and had no experience with the behavior of adolescent girls.

"I don't understand her," he grumbled. "All she seems to do is talk on the telephone about boys and clothes and act silly."

"Why, Ben," I said, "that's not unusual in teenage girls. Most of them grow out of that stage and become intelligent, responsible adults."

"Do you really think so, Gloria?" he asked earnestly.

I smiled. "Ben, can you imagine how strange it feels for me to be giving you advice?"

He referred to our talk in one of his interviews with reporters. They quoted him as saying, "I thought I knew something about adolescence and stepchildren, but it turns out, I don't know B-E-A-N-S!"

Spock's ward rounds with small groups of residents were a particular delight. Few children could resist his charm. He had them laughing and giggling within minutes, not at all afraid of the tall man who loomed over their beds. He listened attentively to the residents' presentation of cases. He occasionally interrupted to question the resident, not so much about diagnosis and treatment, but about how child and parent were coping with the hospitalization. One of the residents referred to a parent as being anxious and overprotective. (These discussions were not held at the child's bedside but in a private conference room.) "Well, doctor," he drawled, "if your child were hospitalized with a serious illness, don't you think you might feel a bit anxious and be overprotective?" It was a lesson I think the residents never forgot. When he left, he gave me a copy of his book, *Baby and Child Care*. He inscribed it, "To Gloria, with Admiration and Love, Ben."

A memorial was held for Ben Spock in a Quaker meetinghouse in Washington after he died on March 17, 1998, and I attended. In addition to his immediate family, the majority of people there had worked with him in the anti-war movement. If there were any physicians present, I didn't know them. The speakers included a son of Dr. Martin Luther King, Jr. Many people rose spontaneously to give testimony after the formal speeches. Most had personal reminiscences to relate and spoke of his anti-war activism. Little was said of his contributions to child care that had influenced the manner in which a whole new generation of children had been raised. I wanted to speak but feared that I was too emotionally involved to sound coherent.

CHAPTER FIFTEEN

Life as Director

B oth Al and I got along well with most of our medical colleagues but I had a significant failing. I found it difficult to tolerate self-importance and pomposity and had an almost uncontrollable urge to needle the offenders. This led to a famous feud with a neurosurgeon, Dr. Joseph K. (not his real name or initial), who had recently joined the staff. He was quite competent but had an exceedingly inflated ego. We started off on the wrong foot almost immediately.

He was a short, heavy man whose belly seemed to lead the way as he strutted onto the pediatric floor one day. He looked around imperiously and focused his gaze on me. We had a census of very sick children, the ward was full, and I was trying to arrange for the discharge of some children who had recovered sufficiently to be cared for at home. We were short-handed and the nurses and residents were scurrying around trying to handle the extra load. I was the only one sitting, making the necessary phone calls at the nurse's station. He stalked up to me and demanded, "Nurse, come with me. I want you to change the dressing on one of my patients so I can examine the surgical incision."

I looked at him mildly and said, "We're short-staffed. Would you mind changing the dressing by yourself? The dressing cart is over there." I pointed to the movable cart that contained all the necessary equipment. He was outraged.

"Are you refusing to follow a doctor's orders?"

"Yes, I guess I am."

"I'm going to report you to the nurses' office."

"You do that. But if you're going to report me," I added, "you'd better know my name. I'm Dr. Schrager, director of pediatrics."

Dr. K turned heel and stalked off the ward. One of his partners changed the dressing later in the day.

Our relationship deteriorated further when I admitted a child who had a stroke. The radiologist and I diagnosed a rare disease of the brain's blood vessels, Moya Moya. The word means "smoke" in Japanese. The Japanese physicians who were the first to diagnose this unusual cause of stroke in adults used that term to describe the delicate, curling appearance of the brain's blood vessels, much like cigarette smoke when viewed by cerebral angiography, a special X-ray technique that visualized the circulatory system of the brain. I was preparing the case to present at our Friday morning conference and invited the radiologist and a member of the neurosurgical department to discuss it. They sent Dr. K.

After the radiologist had demonstrated the X-rays, the neurosurgeon was expected to discuss its significance. Dr. K. was very dismissive. "There's nothing unusual about this case", he said. "I've seen many such cases, and it's been reported in the literature numerous times." "Joe," I said, "I intend to submit this case for publication and I've researched the literature of the past 20 years. I haven't found one report of this condition in children. If you've seen numerous references, I would be very grateful if you would share them with me." He sat down without a word.

The radiologist remained expressionless. After the conference, he took me to one side and said quietly, "I've been waiting for someone to take that guy down a peg. You sure did it neatly."

Our next skirmish occurred when a critically ill child was admitted to the pediatric service as a charity case. The child had been treated for hydrocephalus and had a shunt (a tube) between his brain and his abdomen to drain off the excess fluid that built up in his brain. He was very lethargic and feverish. I feared that the shunt had become blocked and infected. I requested a consultation with the neurosurgeon covering service cases and unfortunately it was Dr. K.

"I know that child well," he said. "I put the shunt in. His father never paid his bill and I told the family I would never look at him again. Send him to the city hospital in Newark."

I said, "The child is much too ill to be transferred. Besides, he is not your private case now. He is a service case and you are responsible today for covering the service."

Dr. K. replied, "Only if he has a neurosurgical problem. I don't believe you are capable of diagnosing an infected shunt."

I snapped, "That will be his diagnosis until you prove me wrong. If you don't want to see him, send one of your partners to cover the service for you."

"Are you interfering with me again?" snarled Dr. K.

"I can't interfere with you if you want to send the father to debtor's prison to rot in chains for the rest of his life," I said. "But I most certainly can interfere if it involves the care of this child. He is not responsible for his father's debts."

"I'm going to report you to the executive committee!" he threatened.

"Oh, Joe," I crooned, "just name the day!"

Another neurosurgeon saw the child and replaced the infected shunt. He said, "It's lucky you didn't transfer him. It would have been very embarrassing for the hospital and could even have led to a lawsuit." The child recovered quickly.

Early every morning I made bedside rounds with the residents and the head nurse, Mrs. Wenzel. Since most of the patients had their own doctors, I would just wave and say, "Hi! How're you doing?" If there was a new problem that the patient, the residents or Mrs. Wenzel wanted to discuss, we would stop and spend more time with the case, but usually rounds focused on the service patients, who had no private doctor. We also reviewed the diagnosis and treatment of all patients who had been admitted in the preceding twenty-four hours. In that way, I knew the status of every patient on the pediatric floor.

We were walking by the bed of one of Dr. K.'s patients, a teen-age boy named Ricky B., whose brain tumor had been surgically removed several days before. His head swathed in bandages, he still managed a weak smile. "I'm doing okay. But could you please get me some more water? My pitcher's empty."

"Sure," I said.

"I don't understand it," said a first year resident, Dr. S., a slim, dark-eyed young woman from India who still preferred to wear the colorful saris of her native country. Her lovely, intelligent face was creased in a puzzled frown. "He still has an IV running for his medication and is getting adequate amounts of fluid. But he keeps drinking pitchers of water."

Mrs. Wenzel shook her head in frustration. "I wish he wouldn't drink so much. The nurses are complaining that he has to urinate every few minutes."

A red light began blinking inside my head. "Let me see his chart, please."

Dr. S. said, "His latest blood tests have just come back and haven't been entered in the chart yet. Do you want to see the results?"

I flipped through the sheets she gave me. His serum sodium level was abnormally high. I said, "Please call Dr. K immediately and give him these results. And tell him about the boy's thirst. Let's go to the conference room. We'll continue rounds in a little while."

Dr. S. joined us a few minutes later, her huge dark eyes wet with tears. "Dr. K was very rude. He wouldn't even listen to what I had to say and told me never to call him at his office. He hung up on me."

I nodded, grim-faced but silent. We finished discussing the reasons for Ricky's strange thirst. The phone rang. It was Dr. K. He roared, "Don't you ever let your residents waste my valuable time again by calling my office! It's bad enough that they get in my way when I'm in the hospital!"

I had difficulty controlling my anger. He had constantly refused to discuss his cases with the residents and he knew that this was an obligation of every doctor in a teaching hospital.

"Oh," I answered sweetly. "I guess I never realized that your time was that valuable. If you can spare some of it, perhaps you can check your patient, Ricky B. He's developed diabetes insipidus. The residents brought it to my attention this morning. If you would spend some of your valuable time listening to them, you might find it helpful."

He slammed the receiver down without another word but came to the hospital a little while later and started the appropriate treatment. Ricky went home after a few more days, no longer interested in pitchers of water.

Diabetes insipidus is totally different from the more common "sugar diabetes," or diabetes mellitus. The only similarity between the two is excessive thirst and urination. Diabetes mellitus is caused by the body's inability to either make or utilize insulin, a hormone produced by special cells in the pancreas, an organ located in the abdomen. Diabetes insipidus (DI) is caused by the body's inability to make or utilize a water-saving hormone known as anti-diuretic hormone (ADH) also called vasopressin. This hormone is secreted by special cells in the brain. Central DI is caused by brain tumor, brain surgery, head injury, or an infection, such as meningitis or encephalitis, that interferes with the brain's ability to produce ADH.

Another form of DI, nephrogenic DI (NDI) is caused by a problem in the kidneys. The brain makes enough ADH but the kidneys, the organs that produce urine and help control the body's water balance, can't utilize it. Sometimes the problem is due to acquired kidney disease. But nephrogenic DI can also be inherited. For example, we had a baby boy admitted to the hospital for unexplained fever. All our tests for infection were negative. I could not find any cause for his fever when I examined him on rounds but I noticed that he was very irritable and appeared dehydrated. "I thought you told me he hasn't had vomiting or diarrhea," I said to the residents. "He hasn't," they echoed in unison.

"Has he been drinking enough fluids?" I asked Mrs. Wenzel.

She answered, "You bet. He drinks his bottle and keeps screaming for more. We have to give him water between feedings but he's never satisfied. And his diaper is always soaked. We change him constantly."

The little red light inside my head began blinking. "Let me see his chart, please."

His serum sodium level was abnormally high. We did the tests that confirmed the diagnosis of NDI. His fever was due to dehydration. I called a pediatric nephrologist to see him in consultation. "I want to speak with both parents," he said. "I want a complete family history. A lot of these cases are inherited."

The parents were an intelligent, pleasant young couple, very anxious about their son's condition. We explained the problem to them, adding, "Sometimes this disorder runs in families. Do any of your relatives have to drink a lot of water?"

They shook their heads. "Our family history isn't going to help you. You see, we adopted Bobby." The mother added, almost as an afterthought, "We went all the way up to Nova Scotia to adopt him." "NOVA SCOTIA!!" the nephrologist and I exclaimed in unison.

There was a theory at the time called "The Hopewell Hypothesis." It suggested that all cases of NDI in North America originated from a group of Ulster Scot who had immigrated to Nova Scotia in 1761 on the ship "Hopewell." This theory was found to be inaccurate when genetic testing revealed that many affected families had genetic mutations different from those of the Hopewell descendents. But Bobby was unquestionably a descendant of the Ulster Scot, and NDI was not uncommon in that ethnic group. In fact, they had a legend that accurately described the inheritance of the disease long before genetics were known. The story, passed from generation to generation, told of a gypsy woman who was traveling with her small son and stopped at a farmhouse to ask for a drink of water. The housewife, fearing that she was a witch, refused to open the door and the little boy began to cry with thirst. The witch put a curse on the house: all the sons of that housewife would suffer from unbearable thirst, and the sons of her daughters would be similarly cursed down through the generations. This is an eerily accurate description of the mode of inheritance of NDI. It is a recessive disorder, linked to the X chromosome. The X and Y chromosomes determine the sex of the unborn child. If the fetus inherits an X chromosome from both her mother and father, she will be a girl. If an X chromosome is inherited from the mother and a Y chromosome is inherited from the father, he will be a boy. The woman who carries the defective gene on one of her X chromosomes is unaffected by the disease because it is recessive and she has a normal X chromosome which dominates the defective one. But 50% of her sons may inherit her defective X chromosome and there is no normal X chromosome to counteract its effect since they have inherited a Y chromosome, rather than an X, from their father. Those sons will have the disorder. The Ulster Scot had figured it out hundreds of years ago.

As the volume of our patients increased, we began to see more unusual conditions in children. We held a clinic each week where residents saw newborn babies whose parents could not afford a private pediatrician. It was the responsibility of the pediatrician on service to supervise the residents and countersign the medical charts of all the babies to indicate that he had personally examined them.

I was in the middle of a meeting in my office when the phone rang. The chief resident, Dr. Arvind Shah, sounded frustrated and upset. "I'm down here in the clinic. Dr. J. just phoned that he has an emergency in his office and won't be able to come to supervise the clinic. We have at least a dozen babies that have to be checked out and I'm really worried about one of them."

"Okay," I said. "I'll cut my meeting short and be down there as soon as possible."

The clinic was in an uproar with crying babies, impatient parents, residents darting from one cubicle to another, trying to cope as best they could until supervision arrived. I rapidly examined the lustily-crying babies and soothed the upset mothers by answering their questions and exclaiming my delight about how well their babies were doing. Relative order was soon restored.

"This last baby is the one I particularly wanted you to check," said Dr. Shah. "He's almost five weeks old and has been vomiting on and off since birth. He's barely regained his birth weight. Dr. J. saw him in clinic last week and arranged for a visiting nurse to go to the home. The mother has a severe post-partum depression and can barely take care of her baby. The father is an alcoholic who seems to have little interest, much less love, for the infant. The visiting nurse has been seeing them every day but the baby looks worse—he's dehydrated and looks shocky to me."

I went into the cubicle. The father confronted me as soon as I entered. He was unshaven, with a few long blond hairs on his chin that I assumed represented his attempt to grow a beard. His greasy blond hair was tied back in a ponytail. He smelled strongly of alcohol, rivaling the odor of his unwashed jeans and T-shirt. Scowling, he used several expletives to express his displeasure at being kept waiting. "And this damned kid has caused me nothing but trouble. The stupid bitch I married can't even take care of him. This ain't my job!"

I ignored him and went to look at the baby. He was emaciated and dehydrated, lying limply on the table, barely able to protest with a weak cry when I examined him. I noted that he had a small scrotum, with undescended testes. His penis was very small. I searched for the urethra (the opening through which urine is excreted). It was not in the usual position at the tip of the penis. I finally found it at the base, near the scrotum. I said to the father, "We have to do some tests on your baby. We'll be back in a minute."

We went to the conference room. Dr. Shah said: "We'd better admit him for IV treatment of his dehydration" I shook my head doubtfully. "Of course we'll admit him and start IV hydration immediately. But I don't think his family is his problem, at least not as far as his illness is concerned. I think that little boy is really a little girl with ambiguous genitalia. We have to do a lot more than correct his, or her, dehydration. But before we call in the endocrinologists, let's get some basic tests done. I'm particularly anxious about the sodium level in the blood. And I want to do some chromosome tests to determine what sex that baby really is."

I asked for stat tests of blood chemistries. Within minutes, the head of the laboratories was on the phone. He shouted, "What in hell is wrong with that baby? We repeated the blood chemistries twice because I couldn't believe the results. They're not the tests of a baby with simple dehydration. His serum sodium is so low it's almost incompatible with life!"

I reassured him. "We've already started IVs that should correct the sodium level. I think that he—uh—she has salt-losing congenital adrenal hyperplasia."

This disorder is usually inherited. It is an autosomal recessive disease, meaning that the defective gene is not only on the X chromosome, as it is in X-linked disorders. Both boys and girls can inherit it. If the defective gene is balanced by a paired gene that is normal they won't have the illness, since the normal member of the pair dominates the recessive member. If both parents are carriers of the defective gene, then the child will show signs of the disease, since there is no normal gene to counteract its effect. If the fetus inherits a defective gene from one parent and a normal gene from the other, the child will be a carrier but will not show signs of the disorder.

The defective gene in congenital adrenal hyperplasia results in a lack of an enzyme that the adrenal gland needs to make steroid hormones. The absence of these hormones, among many other effects, causes the body to lose sodium. This lack also stimulates the adrenal gland to produce abnormally large quantities of another adrenal hormone that does not need the enzyme that is missing because of the defective gene. The hormone is androgen, a male sex hormone. Girl babies with this disorder have external genitalia that may resemble male, although their internal sex organs are female and they can have children once their external genitalia are surgically corrected. Boy babies with this disorder have external male genitalia that are larger than normal but these boys have smaller stature as adults.

Once we had the test results I called an endocrinologist in consultation. He confirmed the diagnosis and recommended treatment to correct the endocrine imbalance. I said, "Now that we're sure, we have to tell the parents. Neither of them has visited the hospital since he—uh—she was admitted. I don't relish the job of telling that father his little boy is really a little girl. He's not a pleasant person—God alone know how he'll react. But we'll have to schedule a meeting and try to explain the baby's problem."

Family dynamics can be very strange. This surly, disinterested, unkempt father brightened considerably when we stammered our explanations. "You doctors sure screwed up," he gloated. "I told my wife all along that we were going to have a little girl! After our crazy wild sons, we wanted a little girl. I'm glad we named him—uh—her Sammy. It can still be Sammy, for Samantha." When we saw the baby several weeks after her discharge she was thriving, dressed in a lovely pink frilly baby dress. Her mother, a shy young woman with long blond hair, was dressed attractively in jeans and a flowered tank top. She was smiling and cuddled her baby protectively in her arms. The father had shaven off his wispy beard and replaced it with a blond moustache that made him look older and more respectable. His hair was sleek and shiny, combed back into a pompadour. The ponytail was gone. He was wearing a colorful madras blazer with navy slacks. He said, "I've gotten a good job now. I'm making good money as a used-car salesman. Got to make enough to take care of my little girl."

There is a tendency when writing memoirs to dwell on one's therapeutic or diagnostic triumphs, but doctors are only human and I've made my share of mistakes. Fortunately, most errors do not cause lasting damage and are soon forgotten by both physician and patient. But a few that I made haunted me for years.

One occurred very early in my practice. A young mother who lived close to our office had put her baby in his crib for his afternoon nap, went to check him, and found him limp, with no signs of life. She ran screaming to the office with the baby in her arms. I was able to resuscitate him, and arranged for immediate hospitalization. Sudden, unexplained fatalities or near-fatalities were known to every pediatrician. They are now called SIDS, the Sudden Infant Death Syndrome. Back then we called them "crib deaths," and they were supposed to be caused by an enlarged thymus gland in the upper chest, a condition called "status thymicolymphaticus." If a child survived an episode of near-death, the recommended treatment was irradiation of the thymus gland. Dr. John Caffey, who founded the new specialty of pediatric radiology at Columbia, totally opposed this theory and warned that irradiation of the thymus could lead to thyroid cancer. I knew Dr. Caffey well. He was a man of strong opinions, and I respected them. But as the youngest pediatrician on the hospital staff in New Jersey, I was obligated to call one of the senior pediatricians in consultation, and he ordered that we irradiate the thymus immediately. I protested feebly, citing Caffey's work, but was ignored and didn't have the courage of my convictions. I still attended Caffey's weekly X-ray conference, and told him what had occurred. He said coldly, "That child was your responsibility. If he ever develops thyroid cancer, you're the one at fault." The boy remained my patient until he was too old to see a pediatrician, and at each visit, I spent an inordinate amount of time checking his neck for enlarged lymph nodes and thyroid lumps. I told his parents that irradiation of the thymus had been found to cause thyroid cancer. He still lives in Westfield, now a hearty, middle-aged man, but each time I see him I make a point of asking, "How're you doing?"

I made another serious error when I was called to see a two-year-old girl who was choking on an unknown foreign body. By the time I reached the house, she had improved, and X-ray examination did not reveal anything abnormal. When she developed fever after about a week, I had forgotten the incident. Her examination was normal and I assumed it was a viral infection. Several days later, she suddenly became septic and went into shock. X-ray revealed mediastinitis, an infection in the middle of her chest, and pneumothorax, a condition that exists when air is in the chest cavity, outside the lung. An emergency operation was performed, and an abscess in the mediastinum was drained. The surgeon found a small, broken piece of plastic jewelry in the abscess. I should have realized that a silent period often occurs after a child aspirates a foreign body, and sometimes an initial X-ray won't reveal anything unusual if the foreign body is not radio-opaque. (made of a material that can not be seen by X-ray.) When she developed fever, I should have arranged for repeat X-ray. She had a very stormy post-operative course, requiring many antibiotics, and developed diarrhea, which continued after her discharge. We tried many different methods to control it, without success. One day, probably due to the thirst associated with mild dehydration, she drank water from the toilet. We were all horrified, but to our amazement, her stools then became normal. I suspect that the bacteria in the toilet water re-established the normal flora in her intestinal tract. She had no further difficulty.

In 1981 we admitted a small infant who looked critically ill. X-rays showed he had a lung infection but all our cultures including TB testing were negative. No antibiotics seemed to help. I finally transferred him to Columbia where they made the diagnosis. He had AIDS; one of the first pediatric cases seen in New Jersey. Unfortunately the state was to see many more. He died at home shortly after he was discharged.

I remember other critically ill infants. During the Vietnam War this country was airlifting Vietnamese orphans for placement in the United States and Europe. A local charitable group in Summit was involved in their care. They requested our services to provide medical backup when the planes arrived at Newark airport and I arranged for one of the senior pediatric residents to accompany the people who met the plane. Most of the children who needed medical care did not require hospitalization. But one day they rushed a very sick, dehydrated infant directly to the hospital. He was in shock and appeared terminally ill. We placed him in intensive care and worked over him for several days before we felt he was out of danger. We could not figure out his age. He was so emaciated that the usual developmental charts were of no help. His motor development was far ahead of his weight but he did not smile or laugh.

A week later he was well on the road to recovery when he broke out in a rash that covered his whole body. It didn't look like any of the childhood infectious diseases and we puzzled over the cause. "It looks like scabies," I murmured, half to myself. "We'd better start treatment for scabies."

Nobody would agree with me. The residents and Mrs. Wenzel said, "He didn't have any signs of scabies when he was admitted. How could he get scabies in the hospital?" Scabies is caused by a tiny parasite, a mite that is almost microscopic in size. It burrows into the skin and causes itching and inflammation. Mrs. Wenzel was particularly incensed by the implication that her ward was infested with scabies mites.

The dermatology consultant thought scabies was so unlikely that there was no point even testing for it. "It's undoubtedly an allergic reaction," he said. I noticed that all the nurses caring for the baby had absentmindedly begun to scratch their hands. On examination, they had the telltale signs of scabies between their fingers. Baby and nurses all tested positive for scabies. We had to institute a mass treatment program. Several months later one of the pediatric journals reported the prevalence of scabies in these Vietnamese children. They noted that many were so sick and malnourished that their immune systems could not react to the presence of the mite until they had recovered.

THE RESULTS OF FUNDING NEW PEDIATRIC PROGRAMS

Page 2   THE WESTFIELD (N.J.) LEADER, THURSDAY, APRIL 24, 1975

Local MD Aids Vietnam Infant Win Fight for Life

A "miracle" story involving a tiny bit of Viet Nam and Overlook Hospital in Summit took place last week.

The subject was a minute, almost lifeless bundle of desperately ill Vietnamese infant.

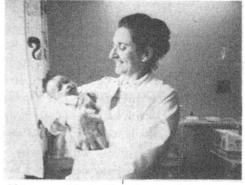

Vietnamese Infant Wins the Overlook Hospital "Oscar"... Alive and well and living at Overlook, is an unknown Viet Nam infant, nicknamed "Oscar" by the Overlook staff. Arriving at Overlook desperately ill with gastroenteritis last week, dehydrated to the point where there was no blood pressure reading, tiny Oscar was rescued by the live-saving measures of Overlook's Pediatric Intensive Care Unit. Here, he is pictured with Dr. Gloria O. Schrager of Westfield, director of pediatric education at Overlook. Soon Oscar will be on his way to his new family in Switzerland.

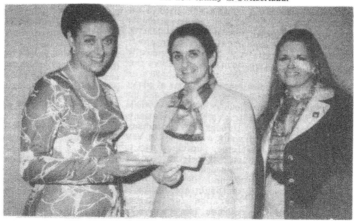

INFANT RESPIRATOR GIFT — Dr. Gloria O. Schrager, head of Pediatrics at Overlook Hospital receives a check for $978.14 from Junior Fortnightly Club president, Mrs. William Wenslau. Looking on is clubmembers Mrs. H. Arthur Cornell who initiated the collection of Betty Crocker cupon sin 1971 to enable the hospital to purchase a Bourne Infant Respirator which has now been completely paid for.

174

As the resident staff became more experienced and competent, I had to respond to fewer emergencies after hours. But a very unusual one happened during the Christmas season in 1980. We had an affiliation with Children's Specialized Hospital (CSH), a pediatric rehabilitation center close to us. Overlook's pediatrics residents rotated through that hospital for training in chronic diseases of children and CSH would send their patients to us when they needed acute care or special testing.

I was just sitting down to a peaceful dinner with the family when the phone rang. "There's been a bomb scare at Children's Specialized. They want to evacuate all the children to us. But all our beds are filled and many of those kids are on respirators— we don't have that many extra respirators!" The nurse in charge, who had called me from Overlook, sounded desperate.

About a dozen phone calls later, a quickly organized evacuation was under way. Many ambulances were mobilized and the children were transported in their beds with their own respirators. The auditorium at Overlook was cleared to make room for an emergency evacuation ward. All residents were called in to assist. Many of the children were very frightened but I noticed a group of Christmas carolers touring the hospital, and I asked them to entertain in the auditorium. We opened the kitchen to supply juice, milk, and cookies, and soon the emergency evacuation had turned into a big party. The bomb scare was a hoax. I could never understand what kind of sick mind would conceive it. Moving those children put them at real risk. Fortunately none of them were seriously harmed by the scare.

One day the ambulance brought us a critically ill adolescent girl in shock. She had a high fever, and was vomiting and complaining of severe abdominal pain. Her father, a pathetic-looking little man in an open-necked white cotton shirt and gray cotton pants, was openly weeping. He seemed to have difficulty understanding English so we couldn't obtain an adequate history of her illness. We started immediate treatment for shock. I did a cursory examination and decided this was a surgical emergency. She might have a ruptured appendix or some other intra-abdominal emergency. I put in an urgent call to a pediatrics surgeon who had recently joined the staff. He was a tall, arrogant young man whose cold blue eyes never smiled. He was one of the very few doctors whose air of self-importance I did not mock. He had earned that sense of importance. We were not good friends but I respected his special knowledge of surgery in children. He came promptly, examined the child and said tersely, "This is not a surgical problem. I suggest you look elsewhere."

Somewhat chagrined, I did a more detailed examination of the patient. I noted that a faint, sunburn-like rash was developing on parts of her body not usually exposed to the sun. A new syndrome had just been reported in the pediatrics literature, and I asked her gently, "Have you been using those new super-absorbent tampons for your menstrual periods?" She was barely conscious but her eyelids fluttered and she muttered, "Uh-huh." She had the toxic shock syndrome caused by bacteria that grow and produce toxins on tampons that are changed infrequently. Her cultures were positive for staphylococcus and we started the appropriate treatment.

Her father hovered around her bedside looking greatly distressed. I put my arm around his thin shoulders to reassure him. Since he appeared to have difficulty understanding English, I explained his daughter's illness in very simple terms. I thought he was a member of the hospital's service personnel or had some other poorly-paying job in the community. My diagnosis was as wrong as was my initial diagnosis of his daughter's illness. He was the CEO of a large international banking conglomerate, and was on a short visit to the United States with his family. When she was discharged he made a large donation to the pediatrics service.

We had another adolescent girl who was admitted to the hospital with an undiagnosed illness. Her parents were going through an angry divorce and she was the center of a battle for custody. She was emotionally upset and began to have stomach pain and diarrhea. She was frequently nauseated, refused to eat proper meals and had lost a lot of weight. She was becoming steadily weaker and more dehydrated. Her private pediatrician, Dr. Kenneth R. admitted her to the hospital for IV hydration. "I may have to call in a psychiatrist," he said. "I've known her since she was a little girl and thought that I could help her with her emotional problems concerning the divorce, but she seems to be getting worse every day."

The diarrhea became increasingly severe and we had difficulty giving her enough IV fluids to make up for the fluid and potassium losses in her stool. Her stool cultures were negative for pathologic bacteria. "Ken, I think we should get a gastroenterologist to look at her," I said.

Dr. R disagreed. "She doesn't need a gastroenterologist, she needs a psychiatrist."

I said, "I've seen a lot of kids develop diarrhea when they're emotionally upset but I've never seen one half as bad as this. It's almost as if she had cholera. I think something else is going on."

"I don't think I could get her parents to agree to any type of consultation," he said. They're tied up in their divorce and it's getting nastier every day."

"I have an idea," I said. "I'll ask one of the pediatric gastroenterologists to give Grand Rounds next Friday and present this case to him during the conference. That way the consultation will be unofficial." He agreed.

The gastroenterologist thought it necessary to do some special abdominal tests of her abdomen, and these revealed that she had a mass in her pancreas. At operation it was found to be a very rare tumor called a Vipoma because it produces large amounts of a substance called vasoactive intestinal peptide (VIP) that causes massive diarrhea. The diarrhea stopped as soon as the tumor was removed.

The pediatrics department at Overlook was growing and becoming well-known in other parts of New Jersey. We were beginning to accept transfers of sick babies from smaller community hospitals. In the late 1980's an ambulance transferred a six-month-old infant because he was becoming progressively weaker and had lost the ability to suck. He had been admitted to the other hospital because of severe constipation and weakness The weakness became more obvious when his eyelids began to droop because he had lost the muscle power to keep them fully opened. His private pediatrician feared that the muscles involved in respiration were rapidly becoming too weak for him to breathe and he might need to be placed on a respirator.

There are many causes for progressive neuromuscular diseases in children. When we discussed his problem with a pediatric neurologist, we narrowed it down to two: infant botulism and congenital myasthenia gravis. We were testing his stools for the presence of the botulism bacteria and its toxin, but those tests took time. The mother insisted she had not given her baby honey, a food found to be associated with botulism in infants. "I want to give him the drugs that will test whether or not he has myasthenia gravis," said the neurologist. "This child is seriously ill and we should try to make the diagnosis and start treatment as quickly as possible."

The parents were reluctant to sign permission for the myasthenia test. "I think my baby looks a little better today," the mother said. "I don't want him to have tests with drugs he doesn't need." I didn't argue or try to persuade her. Mothers have an uncanny way of detecting subtle changes in their babies that others can not see. To me, the baby didn't look better, but he didn't look worse, either. We agreed to hold off testing for a day or so unless the baby's condition deteriorated. I told the residents to call me at any hour day or night if there was a change in his condition. I was still very worried about him.

The following morning I had to attend a meeting at Children's Specialized Hospital and spoke to their pediatric physiatrist, Dr. Marty Diamond, about the case. "I wish there was a quick way to differentiate between botulism, myasthenia and other neuromuscular diseases without doing the neostygmine test," I said. "Stool cultures are taking forever and the family is reluctant to give us permission to test for myasthenia. I'm really worried about the baby."

Dr. Diamond said, "We can differentiate between the two with electromyography and nerve conduction tests. The parents shouldn't object, because the tests are of no danger to the baby and don't involve drugs. If you like, I can do them later today."

"That would be wonderful!" I said. The tests were suggestive of infantile botulism and several days later the stool cultures grew out the organism, *Clostridium botulinum.* The stools were also positive for the botulinum toxin. Our case was one of the first to use electrodiagnosis in this disease and we published the results in one of the medical journals.

The first two cases of infant botulism were described in 1976. Before that time only two forms of botulism were known: the ingestion of botulism toxin from improperly canned foods and the absorption of the toxin from infected wounds. It was not considered possible for infants to either eat or breathe in the inactive bacteria (the spores) and that these spores could become active in the body and produce enough toxin to kill the baby. But we recognized that only very small quantities would be needed: the toxin is extremely powerful. (Botox, now used as a cosmetic, is so extremely diluted that there is little danger of systemic effects.) Infant botulism can only occur in babies under one year. In fact most babies who develop the disease are under six months. That is the reason why honey, which can contain botulinum spores, is not recommended for babies under one year. In older children and adults the spores do not have an opportunity to grow and produce enough toxin to cause harm. The gastrointestinal tract has matured and there are also many more normal bacteria that would inhibit the growth of *Clostridium Botulinum.* The disease can vary from the insidious onset of constipation and weakness with a mild course not requiring hospitalization to a fulminant form that can be mistaken for the sudden infant death syndrome (SIDS.)

Once the diagnosis is made, neither antibiotics nor antitoxin is helpful. The disease must run its course, with good nursing and supportive medical care. We found that a lot of new houses were being built around this baby's home. Botulinum spores are found in dirt and dust and it is probable that the baby breathed in some dust that contained the spores from the construction site. The mother was right: her baby was gradually improving. He required tube feeding because he could not suck but he never became sick enough to need a respirator. It took over a month for him to recover fully. His private physician, Dr. Stanislawa Rosnowski, a former pediatrics resident, and the pediatrics nurses and residents watched him continuously. I was very proud of all of them. We could never have treated the baby without their experienced care.

Because medical care was becoming so specialized, there was a national effort to devise new methods of training residents to care for the patient as a whole, from birth to old age. Bill Minogue was on a committee, sponsored by the federal Department of Health and Human Services, to consider the problem. All the proposals had inherent faults. One day, when Bill had just returned from a committee meeting and a group of us were having lunch, I remarked reflectively, "It seems to me that Al and I arrived at a solution without realizing it. I had special training in Pediatrics and he in Internal Medicine. Together, we could care for the whole family. Being married, we acted as one person: there was no difficulty with communication. Why don't we start a new type of program, where residents are trained in both Pediatrics and Internal Medicine and are eligible to take the specialty boards in both disciplines?"

We applied to the Department of Health and Human Services for a federal grant to initiate a pilot study for a new type of training and we were funded from 1978-1983 at $2.5 million, with Dr. Minogue as principal investigator (PI) for the internal medicine aspects and me the PI for the pediatric part. The program was a huge success and we had our pick of enthusiastic graduates who were attracted to a primary care program that emphasized intensive training in the care of both adults and children. Our new type of residency was featured on the front pages of several of the specialty newspapers—the ones devoted to internal medicine, pediatrics, and family practice. I have had no further contact with the program since retiring, but to my knowledge this option is still popular today.

CHAPTER SIXTEEN

Relations with Columbia and Our Trip to Japan

O ur relations with Columbia became increasingly close and cordial. In 1976, Dr. Richard Behrman, Professor and Chairman of Pediatrics at that time and Dr. Raymond Van de Wiele, Professor and Chairman of OB/Gyn at Columbia came out to Overlook to speak at a statewide conference I organized to discuss recent advances in neonatology and perinatology (the study of pregnancy, labor, and fetal well-being) The meeting also served to publicize our new Neonatal Intensive Care Unit (NICU) and our affiliation with Columbia. Senior pediatric residents from Overlook rotated through Columbia's NICU and were welcomed by Dr. John Driscoll, the director of the NICU at Babies' Hospital at that time. He treated our residents as if they were his own, giving them the training and responsibility that greatly enhanced our program.

Dr. Akira Morishima, Director of Pediatric Endocrinology at Columbia, had been an enthusiastic participant in our teaching program from the start. He visited us frequently to hold conferences and see patients in consultation. He called one day to say he was entertaining some colleagues from Japan and wanted to take them on a tour of Overlook. I was delighted and arranged a special luncheon for them.

I started an extensive communication with one of these Japanese visitors, Dr. Kiyohiko Kato, who was the Director of Pediatrics at Yamanashi University in Japan. He suggested a resident exchange. He wanted his residents to spend several months in our program and have our residents spend several months in his. This was not as impractical as it sounds. American textbooks were used in Japanese medical schools and patient records were written in English. All their doctors were fluent in the English language.

Dr. Kato invited me to go to Japan and give some talks at Yamanashi and Keio Universities. He also wanted to formalize our agreement on the exchange of residents. Al agreed to go with me. He had a special affinity for Asian culture since his tour of duty in the Army, and had brought back many Japanese woodblock prints. There were many places in Japan he had visited that he wanted to show me.

We went to Japan in 1986. Dr. Kato was a wonderful host. Yamanashi University is situated at the base of Mt. Fuji, and the view was breath-taking. Dr. Kato arranged a welcoming banquet for us in a tea house amid beautiful vineyards. As usual, I was the only woman present. The formal Japanese reserve began to melt away as the sake flowed freely. We were all seated on cushions around a low table and everyone was taking pictures of everyone else. I had bought a new camera for the trip and wanted to use it with the flash, but whenever I tried to take a picture it wouldn't respond and then would flash in my face when I turned it around to see what was wrong.

Finally, I handed the camera over to the man sitting next to me, an eminent research professor who had a PhD. as well as an MD degree. "Here," I said, "It's a Japanese camera. Maybe you can figure out what's wrong." He also tried—with the same results. The camera was passed from one person to the next, the general hilarity increasing as the camera stubbornly flashed unexpectedly.

Finally, Al said dryly, "May I see that camera?" It had been set for a timed exposure and once he made the adjustment it behaved itself.

Dr. Kato paid us the great compliment of inviting us for dinner at his home to meet his wife and daughters. They were charming and I was particularly delighted with his younger daughter. I had admired an arrangement of flowers that was artfully placed in front of a Japanese scroll. The younger daughter modestly admitted that she had made the arrangement. "I speak to the flowers," she said in her highly accented English. "I tell them, you are very beooootyfulll but I will make you even more beooootyfulll."

OUR TRAVELS TO JAPAN TO ESTABLISH THE PEDIATRIC RESIDENT EXCHANGE PROGRAM 1986

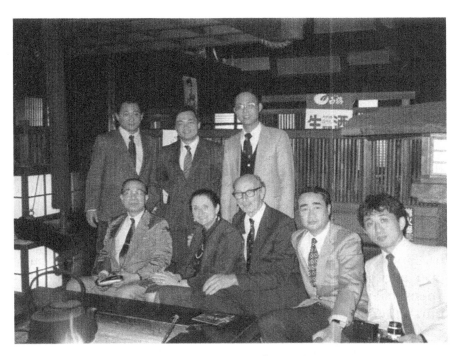

Overlook begins exchange program

Overlook Hospital in Summit has begun an exchange program with Japan.

The story of Overlook's "Japanese" connection began two years ago, when Dr. Gloria Schrager, director of pediatrics and director of the Pediatric Residency Program at Overlook was a guest lecturer at Yamanashi University Medical College, at the invitation of Yamanashi's director of Pediatrics, Dr. Kiyohiko Kato.

During this period, the two pediatricians developed the residency exchange program.

The first "exchange student," Dr. Norihiko Uchida, completed his U.S. pediatric rotation this summer. Uchida has not only added an unusual dimension to his medical education, but has an unusual history for a medical student.

He is 32 years old and had a previous career as a high school physics teacher.

However, Uchida's father is an internist, and his son finally came around to the profession.

He did possess an advantage that a medical student from another country might not have.

"In Japan, we use American textbooks," he said.

"All the physicians in Japan know English. They write their notes in English because they believe it adds to the confidentiality of the patient charts," Schrager noted.

Uchida has returned home to serve on the pediatric staff of a small hospital in Yamanashi, located near Tokyo. But he'll still be in training for another four to five years, to complete his subspecialty area, in a field such as pediatric endocrinology, cardiology, or neonatology.

Afterwards, Uchida will hold the equivalent of a doctor of philosophy, in addition to his medical degree.

As for the "U.S.-Japan" connection, he said, "I hope the program continues forever."

"Several of our residents are considering trips to Japan," said Schrager.

Although the host institution supplies free room and board, travel expenses must be paid by the "exchange" resident.

"Rotations of Overlook residents would be for a one-month period, but would be sufficient to give them a wider perspective of how medicine is practiced in a different culture. We hope to develop similar exchange programs with Italy and Israel, so that our residents can have several options from which to choose.

Dr. Kato took us on tours to various shrines and parks. We even ascended the foothills of Mt. Fuji in a cable car. But we wanted to have some time to tour by ourselves so that Al could show me some of the places he remembered. We arranged to take the bullet train from Tokyo to Kyoto. Since we did not know Japanese, Dr. Kato was apprehensive. He wanted to send a guide with us but we assured him we would manage fine. Kyoto was very beautiful. It was late fall and the leaves were brilliantly-colored. Elaborately coifed and gowned geishas strolled in the evening with their escorts. We were the only Caucasian tourists in sight. Al's height had often drawn attention, but here in Japan it was a particular source of glances and giggles. It was the only place I know where the local inhabitants would be taking pictures of the tourists!

One afternoon we were waiting to be admitted to one of the shrines. Opposite us was a long line of schoolchildren, each group wearing a differently colored little beanie cap to identify their school or class. We could see them laughing and looking at us. Finally one of the little boys, apparently on a dare, came over and gestured imperiously to Al. He barely reached Al's knees. He wanted Al to put his hands out, palms up, in front of him. When Al obeyed, the little boy filled those huge hands with candy and ran away. Al gasped to protest and started forward to return the candy but the little boy was hiding in the group of laughing, jumping children. Al shrugged, slowly unwrapped one of the candies with great ceremony and popped it into his mouth, to squeals of delight.

We flew from Kyoto to Hiroshima. I was particularly anxious to see the memorial to the nuclear holocaust. Standing at Ground Zero was an awesome experience. There was a museum devoted to the history of that event—similar to Yad Vashem, the Holocaust museum in Israel. In one area of the memorial park the remains of a building had been left standing; a mass of twisted steel beams and shattered stone blocks. It was a reminder of the devastation that had occurred. Many school children were visiting the site. They brought with them folded paper birds, cranes with long wings, that they had made. The crane has special significance in Japanese culture as a symbol of luck and long life. They placed their cranes reverently around a memorial to the children who had died in the bombing. I wondered what the other tourists were thinking as they looked at us, the only Caucasians there. "But," murmured Al, "I notice that in their museum, there's no mention of Pearl Harbor."

We stayed overnight at a hotel located near a beautiful park, in Hiroshima. As we strolled through the park, we saw that a ceremony was about to start. Young women in colorful, traditional Japanese dress were arranging an area under the trees. We learned that they had just completed their training in the tea ceremony and as part of their graduation they were required to perform it in front of relatives and guests. One of the older women, a teacher, approached us. She bowed deeply and asked if we would do them the honor of participating in the ceremony. I knelt to receive the tea from a lovely young girl in an exquisitely-designed red and gold kimono tied elaborately with a long, wide sash, the obi. Her hands moved gracefully in the ritual of preparation. It seemed like a form of dance. I was struck by the difference between the beauty and tranquility of this centuries-old custom and the stark tragedy of the city around us.

After our independent tour we were scheduled to visit Keio University in Tokyo. Keio University has the reputation of being the Harvard of Japan. Indeed many of their students and faculty go to Harvard for part of their training. I did not enjoy this visit. I sensed a latent arrogance and thinly-veiled anti-Semitism. One of the young faculty members, recently returned from Harvard, said, "I wonder why there are so many Jews at Harvard."

Al smiled at him benignly and answered, "Probably because Jewish parents are very much like Japanese parents. They both have a great respect for education and want their children to achieve as much learning as possible."

We found Tokyo fascinating, although it did not have the beauty and tranquility of Kyoto. We attended the Kabuki theatre. I never thought I'd see such a spectacle on an enormous indoor stage that was larger than the Metropolitan Opera! Most Kabuki plays are based on well-known legends and can last for many hours. People come and go and many drop in just for their favorite part, often murmuring the lines as the actors recite them. We became so involved in the drama that we stayed much longer

GLORIA O. SCHRAGER, M.D.

TRAVELS TO JAPAN
1986

GROUND ZERO AT HIROSHIMA

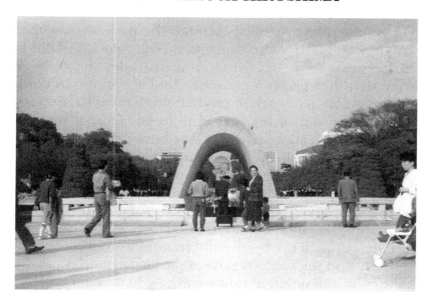

THE TEA CEREMONY AT HIROSHIMA

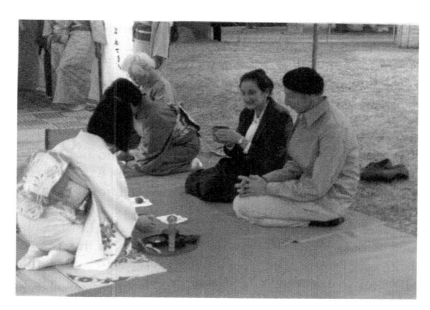

than we planned. Al was particularly excited by a battle scene that portrayed the siege of a castle in the falling snow. It seemed as if many hundreds of people were on stage and the choreography was superb. We couldn't understand the language but we could easily follow the plot because of the stylized pantomime.

We met Dr. Kato again after our Tokyo visit and we started the resident exchange program that we had been planning for so long. The resident staff was delighted and several Yamanashi residents came to our program for a period of training. Unfortunately, I could not find funding for our residents to visit Japan so the exchange was one-way, which was disappointing. Medical standards and training in Japan are at least our equal and I thought it important for residents to see how medicine is practiced in another culture.

Profound changes were occurring at Columbia. Dr. Richard Behrman, Professor and Chairman of the Department of Pediatrics, left to go to Case Western Reserve. He had been a strong supporter of our program. He was replaced by Dr. Michael Katz, who had been doing research at Columbia in infectious disease and parasitology. Dr. Katz's interests and priorities were quite different. He did not want residents from other programs to rotate through Columbia and ordered that they could not have any hands-on experience, even under close supervision. This would have negated the value of such a rotation and I was greatly distressed. I had been sending only senior residents whose ability I trusted and I considered it a vital part of their training.

Dr. John Driscoll, the Director of Neonatology at that time, (he is now Professor and Chairman of the Pediatrics Department) came to my defense and wrote Dr. Katz that the residents I sent were the equal of his own. I was extremely grateful for his support. Dr. Katz also did not look favorably on Columbia faculty going to Overlook to teach and give us the sub-specialty backup we needed, all of which had been stipulated in our affiliation agreement, nor did he approve of the travel to Overlook that took time away from the faculty's Columbia responsibilities.

At an executive meeting one day, I tried to explain how vital their presence was at our hospital. Dr. Katz asked, "Just how far is Overlook from Columbia?"

Somewhat nettled, I answered, "The distance from Columbia to Overlook is precisely the same as the distance from Overlook to Columbia, and if I can come here at least twice a week, Columbia staff should find the time to come to us at least once a month." We kept our Columbia consultants.

Dr. Katz's view of the United States reminded me of the famous New Yorker magazine cover: a detailed map of Manhattan ending at the Hudson River and then a vast wasteland stretching monotonously until one reached the Pacific Ocean. Despite Dr. Katz's somewhat acerbic personality and our occasional skirmishes, we respected each other. Years later, when I retired, he wrote me a lovely letter and informed me that I could retain my faculty rank for as long as I wished.

Dr. L. Stanley James, a perinatologist, was an elegant and distinguished British gentleman. I was greatly in awe of him but found him gracious and ready to help our program with advice, the training of residents, and the continuing medical education of attending physicians. He had been a colleague of Dr. Virginia Apgar, the founder of the Apgar score, and one of the great pioneers in the field. The field of perinatology was still very new, requiring training and expertise in fetal monitoring and neonatal resuscitation.

Many of the older obstetricians at Overlook resisted these advances, and Dr. James was very supportive of my educational programs. He came to Overlook to hold conferences and lend the weight of his prestige to our attempts to initiate these new techniques. He also frequently helped me in my preparations for appearing as a medical expert, of which more in the next chapter. Still, I never felt the easy comradeship with him that I felt with most of the other members of the faculty. It was thus of great surprise when he paid me one of the greatest compliments I was ever to receive. At an executive meeting one day we were talking about the increasing number of court cases charging malpractice. Dr. James was explaining how this particularly impacted on labor and delivery and how at times colleagues you trusted would become unreliable under the stress of litigation. A doctor, instead of defending his management of a case, would blame other doctors for the unfortunate result. Nothing could make a plaintiff's attorney happier. All the attorney would have to do it sit back and watch several doctors destroy each other. It also increased the number of persons who could be sued. Dr. James said, "If I ever get caught in one of these messes, the person I want to defend my back would be Gloria Schrager." I was speechless and turned scarlet. I smiled timidly and nodded in his direction, to show him how much I appreciated his remark.

CHAPTER SEVENTEEN

Medical Expert

$\mathbf{S}$ hortly after I became director in 1972, a lawyer called my office to ask if I would be willing to evaluate a medical malpractice case and be ready to testify for the physician in court. I was reluctant even to consider this commitment. But he was persuasive, and when he explained the charges I agreed that they appeared to be unjustified. Someone should evaluate the case further and be prepared to offer an unbiased opinion. Few physicians wanted to take the time to read the voluminous records that are part of a malpractice suit and then face the stress of a court appearance. I thought, "If we're not going to help our colleagues, who will?" I agreed to evaluate the case and later went to court to testify in defense of the physician involved.

We won the case and other lawyers began to call. Starting in the seventies, I had more cases than I could handle, although I never publicized my interest in testifying. That interest surprised me and it surprised Al even more. "How can you go into court and make yourself the target of that kind of cross-examination?" he asked.

It's true that at first I was extremely nervous but I soon made a reassuring discovery. Even the very best lawyers who prepared carefully and knew all the medical background of a case did not have the clinical judgment to assess the significance of their data. All I had to do was prepare as carefully as they did and I would have the advantage. I also had another advantage. I was an unbiased witness and would not testify unless I believed strongly that what I was saying was correct. And if I could not convince a jury of that after years of teaching residents, something was very wrong indeed.

Being unbiased was the key to the process. Most of the cases I took were in defense of doctors, but if I felt that true negligence or deviation from standards of care had occurred, I would bluntly advise them to settle. I would not defend it. Similarly, I evaluated cases for the plaintiff. If I felt the doctor was not liable for some unfortunate result, I would tell the plaintiff's attorney my opinion that he would probably lose the case. Most attorneys appreciated this: it saved them time and money. When true negligence or malpractice had occurred, I was willing to testify to that effect. Maintaining those principles increased my credibility with both sides.

One of the first lessons I learned was the importance of keeping one's answers simple and not supplying unnecessary information. In one case, a doctor was accused of not properly caring for a newborn infant who had some complications at birth. The plaintiff's attorney opened up a medical book and asked me, "Are you familiar with the writings of Dr. L. Stanley James?"

Of course I knew Dr. James well, had read just about everything he had ever written and used this knowledge to train residents. But all I replied was "Yes."

The attorney asked, "Do you recognize this paragraph?" He then began to quote some of Dr. James' writings that he expected would totally demolish the defense.

I replied, "Yes, I recognize it. I also recognize that you have taken it out of context. Why don't you read the paragraph that follows?"

He closed the book with a snap and changed the subject. We won the case.

I began to enjoy the role of medical witness. Courtrooms are much like theaters, and lawyers are frequently good actors. When you realize that their surprise, shock and indignation are not quite genuine, it becomes more amusing than upsetting. Besides, I had a certain flair for the dramatic myself. I always kept it low-key, but it could be quite effective at times.

Several other cases might serve as examples. In one, the doctor was accused of not taking an adequate history that could have led to the diagnosis. This was manifestly untrue but the plaintiff's attorney was resting his case on it.

"Doctor," he asked me, "when you take a history, don't you immediately determine the chief complaint, the duration of illness, the temperature curve—" he went on and on with a barrage of questions he felt a doctor should ask "—or do you simply say (contempt heavy in his voice) "How are things going?"

"Well, as a matter of fact" I replied, "I often do start an interview by asking, "How are things going? We then have a pleasant conversation during which I find out all the pertinent facts. After all," I said with feeling, "I do not subject my patients to a cross-examination as if they were on a witness stand." The lawyer flushed, the jury laughed, and the judge had to rap for order.

Another case involved the adolescent daughter of a socially prominent family. She had some emotional problems and was under the care of a well-known psychiatrist. When she began to complain of headaches, they were considered emotional but they had her checked by her pediatrician to be sure there was no organic reason. He could find none but suggested performing some tests to be sure. He had recorded this suggestion in the patient's chart. Instead of doing the tests her family took her on a cruise. The headaches became worse and she finally lost consciousness. She was rushed to an emergency room where she died of a brain tumor. The family sued the pediatrician, accusing him of not adequately emphasizing the importance of doing the tests. They recruited a prestigious group of medical experts to testify that if the tumor had been diagnosed and removed, she would have lived. The pediatrician's insurance company offered a large settlement, but the family refused to accept it and the case went to trial.

After testimony by the plaintiff's experts who quoted statistics for survival, I was called to the stand. Helped by skillful questioning from the defense attorney, I explained to the jury that they had to decide whether or not the doctor had adequately stressed the urgency for getting the tests. The doctor claims he did. But even if the tumor had been diagnosed early and surgically removed, I asked them to consider the results of her survival. I explained that the part of the brain invaded by the tumor controlled impulse, emotions and feelings of hunger. I quoted reports that following surgery, many such patients became morbidly obese and were subject to rages and uncontrollable behavior. And there was a distinct possibility that the tumor could recur.

"Survival is one issue," I said. "Quality of life is also important."

The jury's verdict was in favor of the doctor. There was no liability and the insurance company paid nothing.

As I was standing with the defense counsel rejoicing in the jury's verdict, I noticed that the child's father was standing to one side apparently waiting to talk to me. I was reluctant to hear what he had to say but felt that I owed him that courtesy.

He grasped my hands and said, "You know, no one told us what could happen to our little girl if she survived. I think now perhaps we can let her rest in peace. Thank you." He turned away abruptly. Both of us were crying.

I found that many malpractice cases were due to lack of communication between doctor and patient, resulting in misunderstandings. I taught my residents that it was important to keep parents informed and be honest with them about the status of their child. Nothing could be more distressing to a family than to feel that they had no knowledge and no control over what was happening. I stressed the importance of parents' role in giving psychological support and reassurance to their child.

In another case, lack of communication was the fault of the mother. A divorced mother decided to take her children on safari in Africa, even though her divorce settlement stated she could not leave the state with them. When they returned from their travels she neglected to give the children the necessary final week of anti-malarial prophylaxis. One of the children developed a high fever but the mother did not tell her pediatrician of her trip and cautioned her other children to keep it secret. The fever continued despite the usual antibiotic treatment and tests were not helpful. Late one night the child became critically ill, the mother phoned her pediatrician in panic, and he met them in the emergency room of a local hospital. He felt an enlarged spleen (an organ inside the abdomen) and ordered immediate blood tests. The lab technician discovered the malarial parasites in the child's blood cells. The mother confessed that she hadn't mentioned their travels. Since there would be a delay in getting an ambulance, the doctor rushed child and mother in his car to

Babies' Hospital at Columbia. The child had a ruptured spleen (a complication that can occur with malaria). She went into shock and died of internal hemorrhage before they could operate.

The mother sued, stating that the pediatrician was responsible for the child's death. I was particularly incensed by her desire to shift her guilt onto the doctor. Her attorney wanted to paint as sympathetic a picture as possible of a bereaved mother. He said, "You can understand, can't you, Doctor, how much this poor mother wanted her children to have the excitement of seeing lions and elephants?"

I responded dryly, "Most mothers, if they want their children to have this excitement, take them to the Bronx Zoo." The defense won the case.

In general, mutual respect existed between lawyers and medical experts, and I found that we could assist one another in the preparation of a case. There was always the exception, however. One lawyer on cross examination kept referring to me as "Mrs. Schrager." I couldn't understand his motive: was he trying to get me angry, was he trying to undermine my credibility as a medical expert, or could he simply not accept the idea that a woman could have that role? Whatever his motive, it boomeranged. It earned him a rebuke from the judge and the defense attorney used the opportunity to emphasize my medical credentials.

Harassment could take many forms. My normal speaking voice is quite soft and I knew it was necessary for me to speak louder in the court room. But one lawyer on cross-examination kept pacing back and forth, claiming he couldn't hear me and asking me to repeat what I had said. I knew that the repeated interruptions and repetitions were damaging my testimony and I became distressed. The defense lawyer leaped to my assistance. He asked the jury if they could hear me. They all nodded "yes," looking at me sympathetically. He said, "I would suggest to my esteemed colleague that he stand closer to the witness or buy a hearing aid." The jury laughed and applauded despite remonstrances from the judge.

Another lawyer for the plaintiff was an intense, brilliant young man—tall, gaunt, and humorless. He prepared his cases thoroughly and had a well-earned reputation for winning most of them. Pacing back and forth and suddenly firing accusatory or confusing questions on cross-examination, he had been known to terrify medical witnesses into incoherence. We had several cases together that he lost, and it was evident that he was not pleased to see me on still another case. One day he was taking my deposition and asked some questions that could trap me into a seeming inconsistency. I could see where he was heading and eluded him. In exasperation, he said, "Dr. Schrager, what makes you take these cases?"

I replied, "I enjoy the intellectual stimulation, especially (I smiled my most winning smile) when I can fence with *you*, John." He choked, and the lawyer for the defense laughed. "I bet you didn't expect *that* response, John!"

I had some unpleasant moments in the courtroom. I was the medical witness on a case that had been postponed innumerable times. The judge, an irascible old gentleman, finally set a date that he warned everyone would be "firm." Unfortunately it coincided with a time when Al and I had plane reservations to visit France. I told the attorney for the defense of my predicament and she said reassuringly, "The case will be starting just a few days before you're due to come back. The plaintiff always presents first and I'm sure we won't reach the defense until you've returned."

She guessed wrong. The judge kept cutting testimony short with great impatience and they were ready for the defense presentation while I was still in Europe. The attorney had to admit with great embarrassment that I was unavailable. The judge was furious and demanded to see my travel itinerary so he could summon me home at once. He did not believe that the attorney had no idea where I was, and he called my office to speak to my secretary, Dorothy Jeremiah. She confirmed that we had rented a car in France and were traveling without reservations except for the plane from Nice that was to take us home. The judge threatened to take some drastic action if I did not appear in court as soon as I returned.

When we arrived home after midnight, jet-lagged and exhausted, we found a note taped to the door by the attorney:

"URGENT! CALL ME IMMEDIATELY, NO MATTER HOW LATE!" When I reached her by phone, she was almost hysterical. "I've never seen a judge so angry! I know it's after midnight and you have no time to review the case, but I'll pick you up early tomorrow morning and we'll have some time to talk on the way to the courthouse. If I don't have you there as soon as court convenes, we'll be in big trouble!"

I was still in a holiday mood and took the whole matter lightly—a big mistake. I got on the witness stand the next morning with a big smile that was not returned by the judge. He wanted me to respond to questioning by answering "yes" or "no" without discussion and I, used to teaching and explaining, did not take his directives seriously. He suddenly ordered the courtroom cleared. Turning to me on the witness stand he roared, "Young woman, you've given me enough trouble! I make the rules in this courtroom and if you do not obey them, I will find you in contempt of court!"

I was terrified and apologized meekly. When the jury filed back in and saw the change in my responses they looked at me with sympathy, so it came out all right in the end.

One of the cases that I took for the plaintiff involved a month-old infant who had developed a fever. The doctor was a well-trained, conscientious pediatrician who ordered the blood and urine tests recommended for the diagnosis of this problem. But he neglected to order a chest X-ray or a spinal tap. The tests on blood and urine were normal, and there was no response to the antibiotics he was receiving. He reassured the parents that the baby's illness was probably viral. The baby went into a coma and died. Postmortem examination revealed that his little body was riddled with tuberculosis. Cause of death was TB meningitis. The parents were X-rayed and it was found that the father had active TB. He was a merchant seaman who had recently returned from a long voyage and had assumed that his chronic cough was due to heavy smoking. I was extremely sorry for the parents, particularly the father who felt responsible for his son's death. But I also felt sorry for the doctor. He could not forgive himself for not ordering the X-ray and spinal tap on the baby. He pleaded with his malpractice insurance carrier to settle the case out of court as quickly as possible. I tried to comfort him. "Doctors are only human," I said. "With the pressures of a busy practice we all occasionally miss a diagnosis. We're fortunate that the result isn't usually this drastic." A settlement was reached and the case never went to trial.

Another case I took for the plaintiff involved an elderly general practitioner who still performed many procedures that were no longer recommended. He did routine tonsillectomies on most of the children in his practice. There were still reasons why the removal of tonsils and adenoids was necessary but they had to be carefully evaluated by a trained specialist. The child in this case had enlarged tonsils but was not ill very often with colds or sore throats. Seeing the enlarged tonsils, the doctor decided a tonsillectomy was necessary. He did not notice that the child had a deformity of his soft palate. The child developed a severe speech impediment after surgery and the parents sued. The attorney for the defense asserted the tonsillectomy had been done in a skillful manner without complications. There could be no relation between the speech problem and the surgical procedure. I was able to demonstrate with anatomical drawings that the presence of the tonsils and adenoids had compensated for the defect in the soft palate, allowing the child to speak properly. There was no urgent reason for a tonsillectomy but if it had to be done, proper examination of the roof of the mouth was necessary before surgery. Failure to do this was neglect. The jury found in favor of the parents.

I used many of these malpractice cases as examples in teaching residents what to do and what not to do. I found that a simple lecture on do's and dont's didn't hold their attention for long, but once I related it to a specific case, they often remembered it, quoting it back to me, long after.

CHAPTER EIGHTEEN

Bob Heinlein's Retirement and Other Disasters

I t would have been difficult to find a better CEO than Bob Heinlein. He exerted his authority in a firm but pleasant way and was completely trustworthy. Both Bill Minogue and I had given up successful practices and had come to work full-time at Overlook without a contract. We knew that Heinlein's word was his bond. A handshake on an agreement with him was worth more than a bunch of witnessed signatures on a detailed pile of papers. He was not particularly partial to my plans for the expansion of pediatric services and often refused my requests for more funds and programs. But he always gave me a fair hearing and explained his reasons for refusal. I would frequently be frustrated, but never angry. And, with time and persistence, I could often get him to rethink and grant my requests.

I particularly admired his unwavering support of his staff even when we got into difficulty with the Board of Trustees or the community. His secretary phoned me late one afternoon. "Gloria, can you come down here immediately? It's urgent."

Heinlein was sitting in his office with a couple who were well-known in the community. Mr. and Mrs.W. had their lawyer with them and they were obviously very angry. Apparently their infant granddaughter, just a few months old, had been brought to the Emergency Room the previous evening with a broken leg. There was no problem with the care she had received, but the pediatrics resident had reported the case to the Division of Youth and Family Services (DYFS) as possible child abuse. They were threatening to sue the hospital if I did not fire the resident and give them a written apology.

"But she was only doing what she had been trained to do," I protested. "Fractures of the extremities before a child can walk are suspicious for child abuse unless there is some overwhelming evidence of a serious accident—and getting a leg caught in the bars of a crib (the reason given for this injury) isn't one of them. We're not accusing anyone of child abuse, we're just saying the cause has to be investigated further."

Mrs. W. turned on me. "Then you are responsible for this outrage. We're going to sue you for libel. You have ruined our standing in this community."

I lost my temper. "Mrs. W., if you've ever seen a case of child abuse, you would understand why we have to be so vigilant to protect children. I have seen children die because of abuse. And DYFS is extremely discreet in its investigations. If you choose to spread the story among your friends and social clubs we are not responsible for the gossip that ensues. Besides (turning on their lawyer) you know very well that the law protects anyone reporting suspected abuse to DYFS."

The lawyer stood up, and said in a placating voice, "Yes, yes, well, I'm sure we can resolve this matter in an amicable way."

I suddenly regretted my outburst. I murmured some trite platitude that I also wished this to be resolved amicably. As I prepared to leave, I felt miserable. Bob Heinlein had said nothing through the entire episode. At the door, he put his hand on my arm and gave me a reassuring smile. We later learned that the infant's mother had recently separated from her husband and moved in with her parents. She was addicted to drugs and alcohol and had apparently injured the baby while under their influence. The entire incident was resolved quietly.

I liked and admired Bob Heinlein, but our relationship was completely professional. Unfortunately it was to the advantage of certain individuals to spread rumors that it was more than that. This was quite hurtful but there was no way to counteract this gossip.

I discussed it with Al and he laughed. "Hospitals are anthills of rumors. If this makes them happy, let it be. It can't harm us." Al and I had complete trust in each other. Although he had been extremely jealous of the men I had seen before we were married, there was never any question of mistrust since then. We both had ample opportunity for dalliance: he with patients and nurses, I during weekend retreats and conferences. We often teased each other about it. I think it kept our marriage from ever becoming stale.

When Bob Heinlein decided to retire, he called all the directors to his office. He told us that he was going to have the hospital lawyers draw up contracts to protect us when he left. But he urged us to have an independent lawyer review the contracts to be sure they were in our best interest. We told him we didn't think this was necessary, but he insisted. When the lawyer we hired looked at the contracts, he laughed. "I wouldn't dare demand all the safeguards that Heinlein has already put in here to protect you. He's made it almost impossible for anyone to fire any of you without the hospital incurring severe financial penalties."

We knew that it would be difficult for anyone to fill Heinlein's shoes but the series of administrators who followed were particularly inept. None lasted very long. Their only interest was the bottom line, and in pediatrics particularly no more progress was made in medical care or education. We were coasting on the reputation we had achieved, and other hospitals, spurred by our success, had instituted similar programs and were overtaking us. The spirit of cooperation that had existed among the directors was replaced by internecine warfare as each tried to establish influence with the new CEOs. Bill Minogue left for a more favorable position in Maryland.

I found that my access to the front office no longer existed. I had to go through channels, and my written memoranda on the problems faced by the pediatrics program were ignored. The other directors, all men, seemed able to establish more influence with the administration. They all had been able to hire several associate directors to help them run their programs. Despite repeated requests I was denied any assistance and found that the strain of running the program single-handedly was affecting my health.

A new CEO who came from a university center and spoke convincingly of his dedication to medical education and high standards of care, seemed to offer some hope at last. However, I found that his dedication did not extend to pediatrics and he became increasingly annoyed by my Cassandra-like warnings that our residency accreditation was in danger. I began to suffer the petty indignities that corporations devise to rid themselves of unwanted employees.

My office was moved. When I had first come to Overlook, I had been given a large, airy office with many windows, and a generous allowance to equip it any way I liked. I built floor-to-ceiling bookcases along one wall and had bought a large, beautifully proportioned Queen Anne desk and a sofa. After occupying this office for over fifteen years, it was given to the Director of Nursing, and I was moved to a smaller office with a metal desk and bookcases that couldn't hold half my library.

At the annual dinner meeting that year, Al and I automatically went to sit at the table with the other directors and members of administration. The table was still half empty. One of the administrators said, "Sorry, all these seats are taken." The other occupants looked embarrassed and avoided my eyes. I was shocked. No one sitting there said anything, and these were colleagues I had worked with for years! Al took my arm and said, "Come on, Gloria. We've got much better friends elsewhere."

A few days later, I made my decision. "This isn't fun anymore. I won't stay around to see all my work go down the tubes. I'm going to resign."

I went home and wrote a scathing letter of resignation, intending to send copies to the Board of Trustees, etc. etc. Al convinced me that such a letter would be unproductive and it would be more appropriate to retire gracefully "for reasons of health." The pediatrics attending staff was shocked by my sudden decision. They gave me a testimonial dinner attended by many of my friends from Columbia who made flattering speeches. The pediatric staff presented me with a beautiful silver tray. In addition to my name and the date, 1989, it was inscribed, "Beloved physician, Inspiring teacher, Child advocate, from your friends at Overlook Hospital." It was a much more pleasant way to terminate my relationship than my original plan to leave in anger.

Several weeks after the dinner the June graduation ceremony for all the hospital's senior residents took place in the large ballroom of a local country club. When it was my turn to hand out

MY RETIREMENT
1989

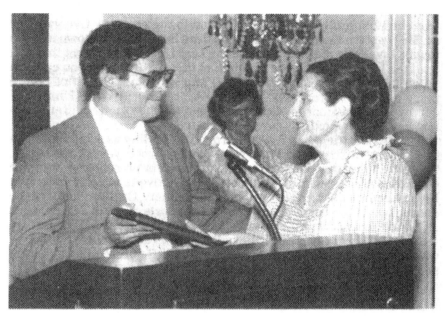

OVERLOOK SALUTES SCHRAGER — Left, Chief Pediatric Resident, Michael Goodman, presents plaque to Dr. Gloria O. Schrager of Westfield, retired Director of Pediatrics at Overlook Hospital in Summit.

the diplomas to the graduating pediatric residents, I realized it was the last time I would be performing this ritual. I was very fond of these young doctors and my voice quavered as I called each in turn to the podium and wished them luck. Several kissed me. People stood up and applauded. A representative from administration made a flowery speech about my service to pediatrics and my retirement. He handed me a huge bouquet of roses. "Be careful," he said, "They still have their thorns."

"How very appropriate," I murmured as I thanked him. There was a scattering of nervous laughter.

The hospital was continuing to expand and the pediatric department was to be relocated in a new wing. I had been poring over the blueprints for more than a year and had many copies made so that I could discuss the plans with the entire pediatrics staff at business meetings. I incorporated valuable suggestions from the staff in my talks with the architects. I pleaded, cajoled, and showed the architects and engineers the plans for pediatrics wings in advanced university centers. I did everything possible to insure that the new ward would have the latest technology and design. The plans included a large playroom, a special adolescent wing with a recreation room, and an intensive-care unit that contained the most modern equipment. There were comfortable facilities for parents to sleep when that was thought advantageous to the child's welfare. The new unit was not finished when I retired. About a year later it was officially opened with much pomp and ceremony. They scheduled special tours conducted by members of the administration. I did not attend and have no idea how many of our original plans were kept in the final version. One of the pediatricians, noting my absence, said to me later, "You're like Moses. You never got to see the Promised Land."

The search committee formed to replace me found that every applicant wanted over double the salary that I had been making. They also wanted the assistance of associate directors and full-time pediatrics subspecialists, requests I had made that had been ignored. Because of our affiliation, Columbia faculty had to be part of the search committee to be sure that the new director met their standards. In order to find a qualified replacement who would consider the position, the administration had to agree to all the demands that I had been fighting for over many years. The person they hired had an impressive CV and came from a prestigious university. The attending pediatricians and the resident staff were not happy with him and his contract was not renewed. It took quite a while for them to find a director who was able to get the program back on track.

I began to see patients again in my old office at home, but had no desire to re-establish a full-time practice, with all its responsibilities. Most of the cases were consultations or second opinions about diagnoses or procedures. I also was able to accept many more medical-legal cases for evaluation and arranged office space so that I could do depositions at home.

Several years after I retired, I learned that the directors of the other major teaching programs (all of them men) were making over twice my salary. Even the associate directors of their programs, young men whom I had trained when they rotated through pediatrics during their residency, had larger salaries.

I decided to institute a suit, charging sexual bias. In addition to the present members of the administration, my lawyer named all past administrators including Bob Heinlein. I asked that his name be removed. I felt that Heinlein would never be unfair. If he had agreed to a salary differential it was because he was following the prevailing philosophy of the time. Married women whose husbands made a good income were considered to be working for the fun of it, like volunteers. If they were paid at all, it was not thought necessary to pay them the same salary as a man in the same position who was considered to be the breadwinner of his family. Looking back now I wonder if Heinlein would have paid me more if I had been a single mother, the sole support of my children. I doubt it.

The hospital offered a small sum to settle and I refused. They wanted to know what sum I would consider. I was so angry I hadn't thought of any monetary amount. My lawyer suggested a relatively modest figure and I agreed. I later learned that I could have gotten much more but my heart wasn't in it. But I had the satisfaction of attending the deposition of the CEO who had caused me such distress. He was thoroughly embarrassed by the searching questions asked by my lawyer. He didn't have a clue about my background and responsibilities. Several years later his contract expired and it was not renewed.

It is important to emphasize that all of this happened many years ago and has no relationship to Overlook today. The entire organization has changed radically. Overlook has now merged with several other hospitals to form Atlantic Health Systems. I barely know any of the present administrators but I am very proud of the hospital's continued excellent reputation. I am still a member of the pediatrics staff, attend meetings and occasionally see patients in consultation.

CHAPTER NINETEEN

Life After Overlook

I had never kept a pocket calendar for appointments during my years at Overlook. Meetings, teaching sessions and the rest of my responsibilities all followed a specific pattern. I had a wonderful secretary, Dorothy Jeremiah, who kept my desk calendar up to date. She would remind me of any alterations in the usual pattern. With retirement, my varied commitments grew so large and confusing that I became totally dependent on my little pocket notebook. It was soon filled with lists, telephone numbers and reminders.

I still had medical privileges at the hospital and did consultations, mostly for my former residents who were now attending pediatricians. I was able to accept more medical-legal cases and found them time-consuming.

A good friend, Melba Nixon, whose children I had cared for when in private practice asked me to join the Board of Directors of the Westfield YM/YWCA, called the Westfield "Y". Melba is an earnest African-American woman who is very involved in community affairs and concerned for the welfare of the children in our town. A dynamic, articulate person, she had become the moving force behind the Y's decision to enlarge their program of child care. I was astonished by her proposal.

"Why would a Christian organization want a Jew on their board?" I asked.

She responded eagerly, "We've become more ecumenical and want the community well-represented. Besides, with our increasing responsibilities for the care of children we would like a pediatrician as a member of our board."

I was aware that there was great need in the community for an agency that could give responsible care to children of all ages.

Westfield had a growing population of families with single parents or two working parents. During my years at Overlook it had been impossible to devote much time to volunteer work in the community and I felt it was time to do that now. I agreed to join the Board and I chaired several committees devoted to children and young adults. The Y not only developed excellent programs for day care, but also for after-school care of older children whose parents had full-time employment. We involved the older children in a host of interesting activities in sports, drama, and handicrafts so that they looked forward to their time at the Y. We even furnished a kitchen where they learned to cook delicious dishes under the supervision of volunteers who were happy to share their family's favorite recipes.

One of the most exciting programs at the Y was the recruitment of a group of mentors: successful members of the community who served as role models, relating one-on-one with a specific child. I can't say we totally eliminated juvenile delinquency in Westfield but I do believe this program was helpful in reducing it significantly. I found that the board consisted of community leaders who were far-sighted, tolerant people who were easy to work with. I enjoyed my years at the Y.

At a medical conference one day, I spoke to Dr. Seymour Charles, a pediatrician in a neighboring community who had been one of the founders of the Physicians for Automotive Safety (PAS). This organization was such a huge success in getting people to accept the idea of car seats for children that it was difficult to remember the time when children in this area were allowed to bounce around a car without restraints. PAS, having accomplished its goal, now had less work to do and Dr. Charles was becoming restive.

"If you want to consider other problems in pediatrics, have you thought about the problems of families with single parents or two working parents?" I asked. We both recognized that grandparents were beginning to assume a larger role in raising their grandchildren, but that frequently disagreements occurred between grandparents and parents concerning methods of child care. We decided to write a book that would address some of these disagreements, discussing both the benefits and dangers of certain folk remedies and the wide latitude of acceptable methods for raising children. We stressed the importance of consistency and lack of conflict among the people involved in the care of a child. When we tried to get our book published we had a discouraging reception. "The market is too small," we were told. "It won't sell."

We finally located an agent who appeared interested. After reading the manuscript, she said, "You'll have to revise this a lot. You've got to make it simpler and more sexy." Neither Seymour nor I had ever talked down to our patients and considered oversimplification insulting to their intelligence. And the idea of writing something more sexy for grandparents seemed bizarre. We had spent a lot of time and research on the book but we abandoned it. Later, several books were published on this subject by other authors and were a great success. They were probably simpler and more sexy than ours.

Retirement gave me the chance to enjoy activities for which I had never had time. I improved my tennis game and prevailed on Al to play with me regularly. He was a natural athlete and doubled up with laughter at my grim determination to win. I never did, of course, but it was fun and my game gradually improved to the point where I could compete on some women's teams and even occasionally give Al a run for his money.

There were so many other activities I enjoyed. What a pleasure to read books and periodicals not devoted exclusively to medicine! And take an early morning swim at the Y. And spend more time gardening—both indoors and out. We had done some renovations on the house and had installed a large garden window in the kitchen. The children had bought me some orchid plants and I found to my delight that they did very well in that environment. There was rarely a time summer or winter that a spray of orchids did not greet us at breakfast.

We had subscriptions to the Metropolitan Opera and the New York City Ballet. As contributors, we could attend rehearsals of the ballet. At one of these I noticed that the man seated a few rows in front, close to the orchestra pit, looked like George Balanchine. Al said, "What would he be doing in the audience?" We soon found out. He suddenly leaped to his feet, stopped the orchestra, went on stage and demonstrated precisely the movements he wanted done. That little episode will always be one of my fondest memories of the ballet.

Another memorable evening was an all-Chopin concert by Artur Rubenstein at Carnegie Hall. When we tried to buy tickets, we found that it was completely sold out. Al would never take "no" for an answer without further exploration. He decided he would try to get tickets a half hour before the performance while I waited in the double-parked car. To my amazement he promptly reappeared with a triumphant grin, waving two tickets. Apparently they had decided at the last minute to allow seating on stage! And so we found ourselves seated just a few feet from the maestro as if he were in our private living room. I had never been a collector of autographs but that evening was so special and Rubenstein's playing so superb that I wanted him to sign our program. We waited patiently at the stage entrance but it had begun to rain and they hurried him quickly into his car. Al decided to write to him, enclosing our program and telling him it would be his fault if we caught cold while waiting in the rain. It was really quite a funny letter and Rubenstein must have enjoyed it because he sent back our program not only with his signature, but with a delightful little note on the side. I have it framed in our study. It says, "To Dr. and Mrs. Alvin Schrager—wishing him a speedy recovery and congratulating him on his good sense of humour. My respects to Mrs. Schrager. Arthur Rubenstein."

With more leisure time I prevailed on Al to take more time off too. We had always enjoyed travel and took several trips each year. In 1991, we hiked the Great Wall of China and visited the terra cotta warriors at Xian. We cruised the Yellow River, saw workers spinning silk at Suchow and bought beautiful scarves for family and friends. We toured Tuscany and expanded our love of art from the Impressionists to the Renaissance painters we grew to know and appreciate in Florence. We stood in awe before Michelangelo's statue of David. Al bought me a beautiful, hand-carved cameo from a shop on the Ponte Vecchio that I still treasure.

Of all the places we visited the one country we kept returning to time and again was France. Despite our profound

LIFE AFTER OVERLOOK

PARIS, 1990

NICE, 1992

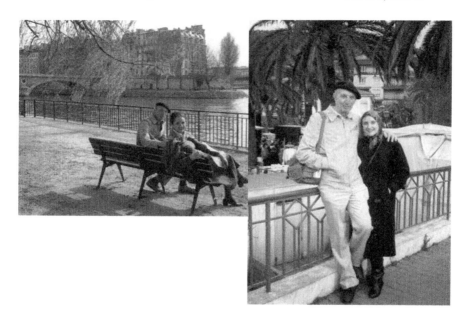

MIAMI, 1991

ISRAEL, 1995

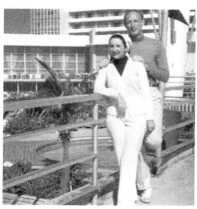
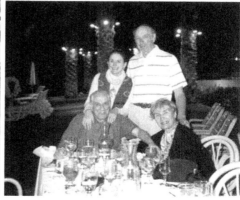

disagreements with French politics, we had a special affinity for the French people. We found them warm and friendly, with a unique zest for life. Al seemed to develop an entirely different persona in France. Usually he was quite formal and dignified with strangers. In France, he wore a beret at a rakish angle and was so good-humored that everyone forgave his atrocious accent when speaking French. I was a bit more fluent so we managed well. We got to know Paris as well as we knew Manhattan. We rented a car and toured the country without any advance plans or reservations. We visited the chateaux on the Loire, hiked through the Massif Central, toured Provence and the Riviera. Al particularly loved the Camargue, the delta of the Rhone river, where it empties into the Mediterranean. Beautiful white horses run wild there and we saw French cowboys rounding them up. There were many flamingoes and I was astonished by their color. They were not the deep orange I was used to seeing in Florida. "I've never seen white flamingoes," I said. Al gave me one of his quizzical looks. "Glor," he said gently, "they're not white, they're pink." It was my color-blindness again! "Well," I said defensively," they're a very light pink." We visited France summer and winter. In some ways, it was like our second home.

Friends of ours at the hospital, a couple who are both surgeons, had returned from a visit to France just before one of our trips. They were recounting their experience, the highlight of which had been lunch at a four-star restaurant. Reservations usually had to be made months in advance but they had been lucky enough to secure cancellations (at a price). The afternoon had cost them hundreds of dollars "but it had been worth it." We were duly impressed but that was not our style.

When we went to France several weeks later, we were wandering through the Marais, a Jewish area close to the Seine. We were tempted by the tantalizing odors from the kosher open-air restaurants. One of them was serving schwarma (lamb and turkey roasted on a spit) and we had them stuff two big pitas with schwarma and vegetables, wrap them up in greasy brown paper, open a bottle of wine, and include a sticky Moroccan dessert. We took the entire mess down to one of the parks that bordered the Seine and had a picnic. It was a glorious spring day. We were just across the river from Notre Dame and sightseeing boats would toot their whistles as they passed. We waved back at the crowds of passengers. Several boys rode by on bikes, gave us the thumbs-up sign and wished us "Bon Appetit— eh?" We responded with a cheery "Merci!" Some American tourists wandered in our direction. They approached us rather tentatively and signaled that they wanted to take our picture.

"Why in the world would you want to do that?" Al asked.

"You speak English without an accent!" said one, amazed.

"What do you expect, we come from New Jersey!"

They looked disappointed. "We thought you were a typical French couple."

Al grinned and whispered to me, "Who do you think enjoyed their lunch more, our friends in their gourmet restaurant several weeks ago or we, picnicking here this afternoon?"

CHAPTER TWENTY

Our Children Grow Up

O ur sons had grown into tall, athletic young men. They both had dark eyes and dark curly hair. Looking at pictures of them during their childhood, it is sometimes difficult for me to distinguish one from the other, though now, as adults, their appearance and personalities are very different. Luke is taller and more intense, although he has his father's marvelous sense of humor. He reminds me very much of Al and is as tall, 6 feet, 4 inches. Ralph is shorter and more easy-going. As a child he was desperately anxious to grow as tall as his father and brother. I looked at his growth chart and promised him he would probably be at least six feet tall when he grew up. He is 5 feet 11 ½ inches and still accuses me, laughingly, of not having kept my promise.

Neither son entered college in the pre-med program. Luke was interested in history and philosophy, Ralph in sports—especially rugby. The one thing Al requested was that they take the minimum amount of science courses to qualify for medical school in case they should desire to apply there. Luke at Johns Hopkins and Ralph at the University of Pennsylvania did well. Luke seemed to be considering law and spent the summer of his junior year as a law clerk in Baltimore. We expected him to apply to law school and were surprised and delighted when he decided on medicine instead. A professor at Johns Hopkins, who was his mentor, strongly recommended the medical school at Vanderbilt University, in Nashville, and he was accepted in1976.

After graduating in 1980, his took his residency in internal medicine at Bellevue Hospital in New York City. His experience there brought back memories of Metropolitan Hospital. Both were overcrowded city hospitals, shabby and poorly-staffed with

MY SONS' CAREERS, 2004

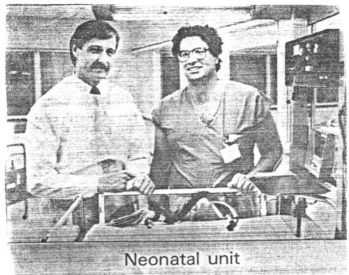

Examining the newly-opened Neonatal Intensive Care Unit at Frankford Hospital's Torresdale Campus are, from left, Robert L. Guthrie, senior vice president, and Ralph Schrager, M.D., head of neonatology.

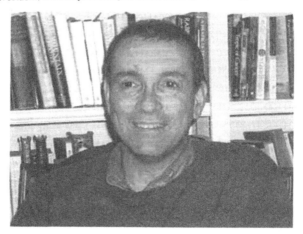

By day, he is a physician in the Federal Drug Agency's Division of Counter Terrorism, and by night he is a writer. "I'm sort of a black sheep [at work]; there aren't any other playwrights," said Lewis Schrager of Bethesda.

His play -Levy's Ghost - is based on real events. It begins on a day in 1857 at Thomas Jefferson's Monticello as main character Uriah Levy is preparing to defend his career before a Naval Board of Inquiry.

support personnel, and both demanded incredible hours of work from their sleep-deprived residents. Little had changed in the generation since Al and I had been in training. Seeing our son go through the same ordeal caused us more distress than when we had been interns ourselves. The realization that he was getting excellent training did not make up for the conditions under which he worked.

A strange type of acquired immunodeficiency had just been recognized among homosexual men. No one knew the cause and Luke became interested in this and other manifestations of infection. He went to Harvard for a fellowship in infectious diseases. While there, the human immunodeficiency virus (HIV) was identified simultaneously by investigators in France and the United States. It was found to be the cause of the acquired immunodeficiency syndrome (AIDS). In the late 1980's Luke did further AIDS research for several years at Montefiore, in the Bronx and then was offered a position at the NIH, the National Institute of Health, in Bethesda, Maryland. In a short time he was promoted to branch chief in the division of epidemiology of the National Institute of Allergy and Infectious Diseases (the NIAID) and continued his AIDS research. During this time he met Frances Marshall, a young lawyer in the Department of Justice, and they married August 16, 1992. A few years later, Luke decided to leave the NIH to do some independent writing. After a while, he joined the FDA, working on a bioterrorism project, but he still pursues his writing career. Two of his plays have been produced. The first, *Levy's Ghost*, is based on the life of Uriah Levy, who bought and restored Monticello, Jefferson's home. It was shown in Baltimore in the summer of 2005. The second, *The Shadow of the Valley*, concerns the Israeli-Palestinian conflict and was produced in St. Paul, Minnesota, in the fall of 2005.

Ralph, our happy-go-lucky son, to all intent and purpose majored in rugby his first year at the University of Pennsylvania. He became increasingly certain that he wanted to be a doctor after he met Debbie Schiller, a pre-medical student, and he began to study more seriously. They were both accepted to medical school at the University of Pennsylvania. Med school is no picnic, but Ralph and Deb seemed to enjoy it more than anyone I know.

LUKE MARRIES FRANCES MARSHALL
AUGUST 16, 1993

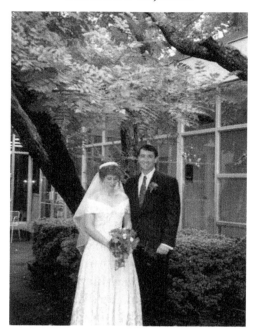

THE NEW YORK TIMES, MONDAY, OCTOBER 10, 1988

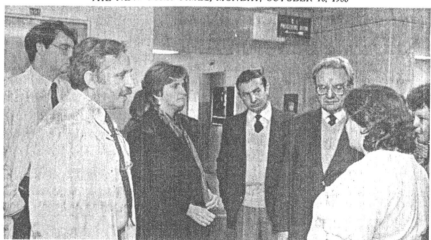

The New York Times/Jim Wilson

Kathleen Eglin, right, head nurse at Montefiore Medical Center's AIDS unit, speaking with Dr. Valentin I. Pokrovsky, second from right, the president of the Soviet Academy of Medical Sciences, who was touring the unit. Also present were Dr. D. A. Orlov, rear, a colleague of Dr. Pokrovsky; an interpreter, and Dr. Lewis Schrager, left, and Dr. Gerald Friedland of the AIDS unit.

RALPH MARRIES DEBBIE SCHILLER
SEPTEMBER 12, 1982

Medical Students Marry At Historic Temple

Deborah Ann Schiller of Flourtown, Pa. and Ralph Matthew Schrager of Westfield were married recently in Philadelphia. Their marriage took place in Congregation Mikveh Israel on the day commemorating the 200th anniversary of the founding of the Congregation, which has been designated a national historical landmark. A reception followed at the Philadelphia Academy of Music.

The bride wore a gown of organza trimmed with Alencon lace and an heirloom train. She carried a bouquet of white orchids and ivy, and a bible which has been in her family for many generations, brought by her grandmother from her birthplace in Ireland.

Her maid of honor was Judith Levenstein, and her bridesmaids were Dr. Alison Binder-Haimes, Amy Levine, Nina Kaleska and Barbara Szczesniak. Best man was Dr. Lewis Schrager, brother of the bridegroom. Ushers were David and Daniel Schiller, brothers of the bride, Seth and Eric Schrager, cousins of the bridegroom, John Kinast and Jeffrey Saunders. The services included selections from the Hebraic liturgy sung by Mme. Nina Kaleska of the Philadelphia Opera Society and Amy Levine, who is associated with the Wolftrap Concert Center in Virginia.

Both bride and bridegroom are senior

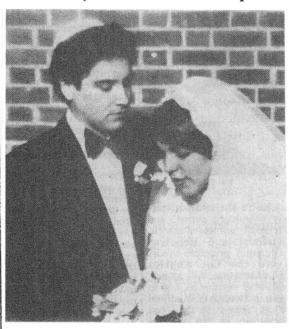

Mr. and Mrs. Ralph Schrager

medical students at the University of Pennsylvania College of Medicine. They will receive their medical degrees in May and will continue their training in Philadelphia: the bride as a resident of obstetrics and gynecology at Pennsylvania Hospital and the bridegroom as a resident in pediatrics at the Children's Hospital of Philadelphia.

The bride is the daughter of Dr. and Mrs. Herbert Schiller of Fourtown. Dr. Schiller practices family medicine in Flourtown and Roxborough, Pa. His wife, Ruth Schiller, is director of services for senior citizens with the YM-YWHA of Philadelphia.

The bridegroom is the son of Drs. Alvin and Gloria Schrager, of Westfield. Dr. Alvin Schrager practices internal medicine and is a former chief of the Department of Internal Medicine at Overlook Hospital in Summit. His wife, Dr. Gloria Schrager, is director of pediatrics at Overlook Hospital and associate clinical professor of pediatrics at the Columbia University College of Physicians and Surgeons.

Debbie has a lovely voice and starred in many of the school's musical productions. She even convinced Ralph to join the cast of "Guys and Dolls." The dean of the college at that time, Frederick Burg, was Officer Brannigan in that play. Their easy relationship was profoundly different from my experiences in med school!

I will never forget Debbie's first visit to our house. They came for the weekend, arriving very late Friday night after an exhausting day in classes and labs. Debbie, overwhelmed with fatigue and nervousness became sick in the car. She entered the house, disheveled and miserable, and made straight for the shower and bed. The next morning she came down to breakfast looking shy and apologetic. Al looked up from his grapefruit and said cheerfully, "Why, good morning, Miss Nausea!" Debbie began to giggle. She had a naturally effervescent personality with a ready smile and had short blond hair that bounced when she walked. Her friendly manner and sparkling eyes won us over immediately. Her meeting with Al that morning was the start of a beautiful friendship.

In 1982, during their senior year in med school, Debbie and Ralph were married in Mikveh Israel, a synagogue whose history goes back to colonial times. It is located just a block from Independence Hall and the Liberty Bell in downtown Philadelphia. Among its prized possessions are letters of greeting from George Washington and other colonial leaders. Rabbi Toledano was a charming man with warm, humorous dark eyes. We felt like old friends as soon as we met him. He conducted the ceremony in the Sephardic tradition, wearing a top hat and white gloves in addition to the rabbinic vestments. Al and I, who are from another branch of Judaism, the Ashkenazim, were enchanted. The synagogue itself, built along simple, classic lines, was one of the most beautiful I had ever seen. The Sephardic branch of Judaism are descendants of Jews who settled along the Mediterranean basin, in Spain, Italy, Greece, Turkey, the Middle East and northern Africa. The Ashkenazim are descendants of Jews who settled in northern Europe in places like Russia, Poland, Germany and the Scandinavian countries. The Jewish population of the British Isles is mixed. Many Jews escaping the Spanish Inquisition found refuge in the

Netherlands, noted for its religious tolerance, and from there migrated to Great Britain, encouraged by Oliver Cromwell, who recognized their value as a Spanish-speaking people who were hostile to Spain. They could help him in his struggles with that country.

Ralph continued with a residency in pediatrics and then a fellowship in neonatology at the Children's Hospital of Pennsylvania (CHOP). Debbie decided to specialize in obstetrics and gynecology and accepted a residency at Pennsylvania Hospital. Ralph then became Chairman of Neonatology at Frankford-Torresdale Hospital in north Philadelphia. Debbie is in OB/GYN private practice.

The summer that Luke and Frances were to have their wedding, we had already made reservations for a short vacation in France. Being involved with wedding plans, I was somewhat reluctant to go. But Al was insistent. "I want to buy them a French antique desk as a wedding present," he said. We had several French antiques at home and we knew that Luke had always enjoyed studying at one of the desks. Al had been scouring the antique markets near us for months but the prices were prohibitive.

I told Al he was out of his mind. "The rate of exchange is very unfavorable. And consider the shipping charges. Even if we find something we could afford, the extra costs would make it impractical."

When we went to France, Al stubbornly persisted in checking all the antique shops on the Left Bank. We found just what we wanted in one of them. I looked at the price tag, mentally converting the francs to dollars. "This would cost something over $25,000," I murmured.

Al began to laugh. "You must have misplaced the decimal."

The dealer also laughed. "Of course you are mistaken, Madame." He busied himself on his computer and finally looked up apologetically, "Oui, Madame, you are correct. It would cost something in excess of $25,000 in American money."

Al would not give up. There is an area in Paris that has flea markets and also antique shops that are open only on weekends. He dragged me from one antique shop to another. We found a few desks that might have been satisfactory but the prices were very high. I suspected that some were reproductions. Hot, tired and losing patience, I sat down on a bench in the shade of a locust tree and said, "I've had enough. This is a wild-goose chase."

Al went to an open-air cafe and ordered cool drinks for both of us. "You stay here and rest a while," he said. "I'm going to look around a bit longer."

He came back about a half hour later. "I've found it!" he called triumphantly. He led me to an alley where a little old man, whose gray, bushy moustache almost hid his ingratiating smile, was selling all kinds of disreputable old trinkets and postcards. A huge red neckerchief added a spot of color to his faded blue smock. I exclaimed in English, while he looked on, uncomprehending, "But this is just junk!" "Yes, but look what the junk is resting on", said Al.

Under the cheap, touristy baubles was an antique desk whose exquisite carving and golden filigree could barely be seen through layers of dust. Al began the traditional bargaining ritual: he said the desk was old and battered but as a favor we would take it off his hands. The dealer began his part of the ritual: it had been in his family for centuries and it would break his heart to part with it. They eventually struck an agreement, the price much less than we had ever hoped to pay.

But how to ship it to JFK? I had a sudden inspiration. Neither of us had checked any luggage. We always traveled light with just carry-on bags. I called the airline and asked if we could check the desk in lieu of our luggage allotment. The airline official hesitated a moment, then said it was a bit unusual but that the weight of the desk would be approximately the same as the maximum amount allowed for the weight of our combined luggage. He gave us his name and said, "Ask for me when you check in. I'll see that you don't have any difficulty."

We entered into a long discussion with our little friend about payment. He declared that he loved Al like a brother, but we would have to pay him in advance if he were to deliver the desk to the airport the next day. We said we trusted him like family, but it was too much to expect us to pay the entire amount before receiving delivery of the desk. We finally agreed on half the amount now, the other half at the airport the following day. I went to the nearest ATM and drew out the required amount, still a hefty sum. He kissed us on both cheeks and bid us "À Demain"—until tomorrow.

As we waved goodbye Al murmured, "I wonder if we will ever see our affectionate friend or that desk again."

I couldn't sleep that night. Although the price we had paid was almost too good to be true, it still would be a lot of money to lose if the desk never showed up. I then had even more frightening thoughts. What if we were the unwitting couriers of contraband—drugs, or worse still, a bomb?

At the airport the next day, we asked for the airline official we had spoken to. He greeted us, looked around, and asked, "Where is the desk?" We smiled weakly and said it was on its way. The first boarding call—no desk. We were becoming anxious when we saw, rolling towards us as if under its own power, a huge object that extended in all directions from the top of a luggage cart. It was sloppily wrapped in brown paper with lots of rope. Peering out from the other end, unable to see over the top, was our friend. He apologized profusely for being late. We paid him the remaining money and bid him a fond farewell.

I alerted the airline official, who took us through customs and security. When the security official asked the usual questions, I responded truthfully. No, I did not have the address of the seller; No, I had not seen it wrapped; No I didn't know what was in the desk drawers. "I hope you will examine it thoroughly," I said, "for our protection and the protection of all the other passengers."

He responded with a typical Gallic shrug. "Do not worry yourself, Madame," he said gallantly. "We will take care of it."

When we reached JFK, the next problem was how to get the desk home. Al did not trust a commercial mover and decided to put the desk on the top of our car. We had left it in the long-term parking lot. The airline officials were again extremely helpful. I think they were all amused by our cumbersome and unusual burden. They got a group of men to lift it onto the roof of the car and secure it with ropes they passed through the open windows in the back. The desk was on its back with legs sticking straight up in the air. It had a decidedly odd appearance and many people stopped to stare and offer comments, advice, jokes, and criticism. After all, they were New Yorkers! We smiled good-naturedly.

We found that the car with desk on top could not fit in any garage. "What are we going to do now?" I asked. "The wedding is not until next week, there is no way to protect it from the rain the way it is wrapped and it would be some job to take it off the car and have to put it back on."

"There is only one solution," said Al. "We'll take it down to Maryland today."

He was too excited about his purchase for me even to think of arguing.

We called Luke and Frances and told them we had just returned from France and had bought their wedding gift there. We were going to take a little nap after our travels and then drive immediately to Maryland to deliver it.

When we arrived they were speechless. Frances had some French cousins and friends staying at their home for the wedding. They all helped us unload the desk and move it to the living room. One of the men worked for the French ministry of culture and looked at the desk with a critical eye. "You know," he said quietly, "this desk is of museum quality." It still stands in their living room, after being restored to mint condition. Whenever I go to visit, I think of how we obtained it.

We went home and returned a week later for the wedding. Luke and Frances, both tall, made an unusually attractive couple. With our combined families, many states, countries, and religions (or lack thereof) were represented, but everyone danced happily to a Klezmer band. Al and I looked at each other. It was good to have both our sons happily married at last.

CHAPTER TWENTY-ONE

Ralph's Illness

A t the end of 1992 we planned to celebrate New Year's Eve together with friends at Luke and Frances' home. I was concerned because Ralph had developed a bad cough and I didn't know whether he would be well enough to travel to Maryland. Luke assured us that he and his family were on their way. The weather was very mild, and Luke had decorated their back patio with colored lights for dancing and a buffet. It was all very festive and everyone seemed in high spirits.

When Ralph arrived, he and Luke said they wanted to speak with Al and me in one of the upstairs bedrooms. They told us that Ralph had just been diagnosed with Hodgkin's Disease, a form of cancer, and would be entering the hospital for treatment after New Year's Day. All the guests downstairs knew and were prepared to leave if we couldn't face an evening of company.

"Of course we'll celebrate New Year's Eve together," I said. "The kids have been looking forward to it for weeks, and have gotten all the silly paper hats and noisemakers. They've even been rehearsing a skit for us."

Smiling, we all applauded the children's performance and I danced with my husband and my sons. We ushered in the New Year with champagne and song. When we left the next day, we waved the usual cheery goodbye and honked our horn. As soon as we were out of sight I lost control and began to sob. I heard a muffled groan and Al pulled the car to the side of the road. It was the only time I had ever seen him cry. We clung to each other until we both regained some semblance of composure.

The following several years were a nightmare. Ralph seemed to respond initially to chemotherapy and went into remission but he had a recurrence and had to be hospitalized for more

DEBBIE'S ARTICLE DURING RALPH'S ILLNESS
ALUMNI NEWS, PENNSYLVANIA HOSPITAL, 1994

MAKING A DIFFERENCE

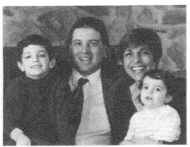

Joshua, Ralph, Debbie, and Benjamin Schraeger

I met my husband the first day of my freshman year in college. We got married in medical school (where we were cadaver partners!) and went on to be placed through the Couples Match in two fine programs in Philadelphia. We both were lucky enough to get our first programs of choice: I ended up as a resident at Pennsylvania Hospital and my husband Ralph, now a neonatologist, ended up at Children's Hospital.

I really enjoyed my residency. I felt very supported having a husband going through the same experience at the same time. We developed a group of friends, who to this day, remain close to us.

Pennsylvania Hospital was a stimulating place to be for a young resident. The senior residents were excellent teachers, many of whom have now gone on to be fairly prominent people. I feel fortunate to have had the opportunity to know them and learn from them.

I decided to stay on at Pennsylvania Hospital and join its obstetrical staff in part because of the excellent quality of the resident training program in which I have continued my involvement as part of the attending staff. Knowing Pennsylvania Hospital had both good support services and an excellent medical staff made the decision even easier. I also knew it was a great place to have a baby since I had delivered my two children here. In short, I felt I could continue my education as well as practice obstetrical medicine in a premier setting.

I have watched the residency training program change over the years from Dr. Wallach's initial leadership, which gave the program its founding vitality and strength, to the innovation which continues under Dr. Woodland's dedication and energy. Dr. Woodland's increased emphasis on didactic education, together with features such as Grand Rounds and The Journal Club, has created an even more well-rounded program.

Pennsylvania Hospital has also been an innovative and responsive institution for me professionally. When my five-female group practice needed to regroup due to the changes in health care, Pennsylvania Hospital agreed to a joint venture with us.

This new venture supports us with resources such as marketing, group benefits, and contract negotiation while we remain independent and fiscally responsible for our success. The Hospital in turn will target primary care to bring more patients into its system.

The many people I have met at Pennsylvania Hospital over the years have reached out to support both Ralph and me during his battle with cancer. My husband, who was diagnosed more than a year ago with Hodgkins Lymphoma, is known to many both from his Fellowship here and as current Director of the Neonatal Intensive Care Nursery at Frankford Hospital.

He has continued to work full time even through chemotherapy and the subsequent remission. Recently diagnosed with a recurrence, Ralph recently underwent a bone marrow transplant. I admire his stamina and courage. I also appreciate the care and kindness of the staff. Hardly a day goes by when someone—physicians, residents, nurses, and even housekeeping staff—does not stop me and inquire about his health.

Balancing this challenge together with the care of our children Joshua (6) and Benjamin (2), a full-time private practice, and serving as an attending physician takes some doing. It has been the day-to-day care of patients that has anchored me. Especially through the last year, the support I have received from patients is rewarding.

As I deliver my patients' second and third babies, I get to know their families and the problems they have more intimately. Having been through the birthing process myself, I have a new respect for both labor and the life changes that follow. As an obstetrician, caring for women who are truly interested in their health and good preventive care during pregnancy gives me the opportunity to really make a difference in their lives. ◆

aggressive treatment. He had total body radiation followed by bone marrow rescue and additional chemotherapy. He lost his beautiful curly black hair and became completely bald.

We went to see him at the hospital the weekend following his radiation treatment. I had made a picnic lunch. It was a beautiful spring day and I thought that if he were well enough perhaps we could eat outside on the hospital grounds. His oncologist, a good friend, said, "Sure. It will be several days before the radiation takes effect. Ralph, you can even go home for several hours if you wish."

Josh (Ralph and Deb's older son) was playing in a Little League baseball game, and Ralph had been a coach. We went to see the game. Ralph even pitched a few innings and then we all picnicked together in the park. Josh looked at his father hopefully. "Dad, can you come home now?" he asked.

"No," said Ralph. "But I'll be home pretty soon. You know, it's a lot like being on call. I have to be at the hospital for a while, but I'll be home before you know it."

My picnic lunch stuck in my throat, and I turned away to hide the tears.

Ralph had his bone marrow transplant the following week. He had to be in isolation and developed some of the complications that occur when the immune system is depressed by radiation. He had a severe case of herpes zoster (shingles) and monilial (yeast) infection in the mouth and throat. It was difficult for him to eat but I made special dishes that he had always loved and brought them to the hospital on our frequent visits. He said that despite the pain he looked forward to this food and it helped sustain him.

It is difficult to explain the feelings of a parent faced with the critical illness of a child. As a physician offering comfort and support, I had been through this experience with patients but now I was on the other side of the fence. I had always empathized with parents' anxieties but felt for the first time the desperate fear, the frustration, the anger and helplessness that assault them. Parents spend many years nourishing and protecting their children. To suddenly find a child in great danger and to be powerless to help despite every instinct screaming "DO

SOMETHING!!!" is one of the most dreadful experiences a parent can face.

When we visited Ralph we were always upbeat and cheerful. Debbie made this even easier. She was incredibly courageous, dealing with the anxieties of their sons in a very positive, matter-of-fact way. Josh and Ben missed their father greatly. Deb was quite honest with them, telling them he had cancer but that the treatment he was getting at the hospital should make it disappear so that he could come home soon.

It was only in the privacy of her bedroom that we let the mask fall and spoke openly of our feelings. We had always been close but sharing our concerns and supporting each other formed strong bonds of love that are not usually seen in a relationship with a daughter-in-law. The entire family seemed to draw closer as if together we could fight off the evils that threatened. Luke and Frances visited often. Luke had always expressed his affection for Ralph with a long string of insults, and having him continue this practice seemed to bring a degree of normalcy into our life.

An ardent fly fisherman, Ralph spent his time in isolation making beautiful flies with a special kit. "When I'm over this," he told his brother, "I'm going to go fishing with these flies in Alaska."

Luke, who didn't enjoy fishing at all, said, "And I'll go with you."

Ralph brightened considerably. "It's a date!" he said. When Ralph was ready to be discharged, he went back to work immediately in the NICU at Frankford-Torresdale. The only time he missed was the one day a week when he received maintenance chemotherapy. It caused severe nausea and malaise. Medication relieved the side effects somewhat but it still was not pleasant. Some of his college friends offered to bring him marijuana which is more effective than most of the drugs approved for the nausea of chemotherapy. We never discussed whether he accepted the offer. He found that he could go home to bed and feel miserable, or he could go out and play golf. The latter seemed to help take his mind off his discomfort and his game improved considerably. His partners remarked that this was indeed a strange way of improving one's golf.

His hair grew back rapidly once he finished his course of chemotherapy, though it never regained the wonderful curl that I loved. Within a year, it would have been difficult for anyone to determine that he had been seriously ill. His oncologist was sure that his positive attitude had helped with his quick recovery and asked him to speak to several young people who were going through the same ordeal. He was of course glad to do this. I was very proud that my son had the capacity to help people, not only as a physician, but also as a human being. Luke and Ralph did indeed go fishing in Alaska several years later. Luke kept a journal of the trip. It was both humorous and touching. I hope he will publish it some day.

CHAPTER TWENTY-TWO

Al's Death

In the spring of 1995 we toured Israel with our good friends, Charlie and Ros Neustein. We had a wonderful visit. During the last week we went to Jordan. We visited Petra, which I consider one of the wonders of the world, with huge ancient buildings carved into the many-colored rock. To get to the ruins it is necessary to go through a long, narrow canyon. You can hike through, go by pony cart, or ride horseback. I noticed that the horses were quite spirited. Although they would amble along docilely, led by their young handlers when tourists were in the saddle, they would gallop at great speed when returning from the ruins with their handlers on their backs. I paid to ride without being led, and trotted happily through the canyon, with Al laughing and striding rapidly after me. We spent the day exploring the ruins and hiking up the steep slopes. By late afternoon, everyone looked hot and tired—except Al. He never seemed to show signs of physical discomfort.

On the trip home we talked quietly about re-entry. For once, we did not have any pressing problems waiting for us at home. Al stretched out contentedly. "You know, Glor," he said, "Ralph seems to be recovering nicely and is back to work. Both boys are happily married and we can be proud of their careers. They've given us wonderful grandchildren. I think we can finally settle down and lead normal lives."

Five days later, on Wednesday, May 17, 1995, Al went to morning prayers at the synagogue as usual. When he returned, we had breakfast and he said he was going up to Overlook for a short while. "It's your day off," I protested. "We have an appointment to play tennis."

Al said he had to catch up on a lot of things after his vacation but would be back in plenty of time for our tennis game. About an hour or so later, the hospital called. He had had a massive heart attack and had been rushed to Morristown Memorial Hospital for emergency heart surgery.

I couldn't reach either of my sons. Luke was at a meeting in California and Ralph and Deb were on their way to visit some friends in New Jersey. Fortunately, their housekeeper knew where they were going. I left a half-coherent message with their friends and drove wildly to Morristown. That hospital is unfamiliar to me and it took a while to explain to the people at the information desk why I was there. I had the eerie feeling of being out of control—not the confident professional on home territory, but the anxious relative in strange surroundings, waiting for news of a loved one.

They showed me to a waiting room. After what seemed an eternity, the cardiologist, Dr. Greg Sachs, a good friend of Al's, came in, ashen-faced. He told me that the surgeons were doing everything they could but the prognosis was grave. He was going back to the OR and would let me know the outcome as soon as possible.

I had never felt so helpless and alone, sitting there quietly, just staring into space. To my great relief, Ralph and Deb suddenly appeared. They had phoned their friends from their car to get directions to their house, had gotten my message and altered their course to drive directly to Morristown. It felt good to have part of my family with me. In a short time, Dr. Sachs returned. I could tell from his expression what the news would be.

"He didn't make it," he said quietly.

"My God," I said and buried my head in Ralph's shoulder. I could hear Deb weeping as she leaned close to us. For some reason I couldn't cry. Looking up, I saw Greg Sachs close to tears. Unaccountably, I felt I had to comfort them all.

After quietly deciding what arrangements had to be made, we went back to the parking lot. I automatically headed for my car. "Mom, you're not going to drive back alone," Ralph said. "You're going to come with us in our car."

I protested, "I'm perfectly capable of driving my car. We can't just leave it here."

"We'll worry about that later," Ralph said. "For our sake, please come with us. I want us to be together."

The news spread rapidly through Overlook. We were scarcely home when Carolkay Lissenden called to ask what she could do. I told her about the deserted car in Morristown and she said that she and her husband, Bart Barre, would drive out immediately to pick it up. When they came by to pick up the keys, I realized the comfort of having such good friends.

I had no idea how we could reach Luke. All I knew was that he was speaking at a conference at one of the California universities. Ralph said quietly, "I'll find him", and he did. Luke took the next plane home.

Funeral services were held at the synagogue. The entire building was packed with family, friends, medical colleagues, and patients. We were in seclusion in the rabbi's study before services started. There was a soft knock on the door and someone put his head in and said apologetically, "There is a man out here who says it's extremely urgent to speak with you." We nodded, and he ushered in a distraught, elderly man who looked at us accusingly.

He said querulously, "I had an appointment to see Dr. Schrager this afternoon. It was very important. What am I supposed to do now?"

Luke gently ushered him out, reassuring him that other doctors would be caring for Al's patients. We looked at one another helplessly and suddenly burst into hysterical laughter. With tears running down her cheeks, Debbie gasped, "Dad did that. He wanted us to laugh at his funeral."

Both my sons, Rabbi Zell, and several friends and colleagues spoke very movingly at the services. I was determined not to lose control, refused any assistance, and moved quietly through the ordeal at the burial. When people came up to express condolences many were crying but I was not. Frankly, I think I was just too numb with shock.

The reaction set in after the period of shiva, the days following the funeral, when a Jewish family sits at home together and receives visitors who join in the prayers for the deceased. My sons wanted me to go home with one of them but I refused. I knew it was important to re-establish my own life and not be dependent on anyone. Still, being alone in that large empty house was almost unbearable.

I had never realized the severe, crushing horror of emotional pain with no one to share it. Our wedding anniversary was the following week, then Father's Day and Al's birthday a few weeks later. I went back to the cemetery and screamed at him. "How dare you do this to me?" Then I wailed like a banshee in the deserted cemetery. I suddenly remembered Dr. Wilhelm Reich, Eva's father, talking about the primal scream which was supposed to relieve emotional tensions. I did not find this to be true. These episodes left me exhausted and more depressed than ever.

I felt that a vital part of me had been amputated and that I could not go on living with such a disability. I had enough insight to realize I needed psychiatric help. Eve Wood, a dear friend who is a psychiatrist, talked with me and was a very great comfort. She put me on a mild antidepressant which was helpful, but I think exercise was even more effective.

I would wake at about five each morning, unable to get back to sleep. The dark and the loneliness pressed in on me. It seemed impossible to get out of bed, much less face the day. I forced myself up and into a swim suit. The indoor pool at the JCC, the Jewish Community Center in Scotch Plains, a neighboring community, opened at 6:30 AM and I was there as the door opened. I swam a full mile each morning and then worked out in the gym. By then I was exhausted and even a bit hungry. After breakfast there was work to do, and so the days passed.

Gradually things began to improve. I would still have sudden episodes of unbearable grief brought on by unexpected sights or sounds—seeing the porch swing Al had bought me for a birthday, where we had sat and talked on many summer evenings, hearing a song or even a phrase someone would say that would awaken memories. When I heard a car door slam, I would automatically think, "He's home at last." These episodes were painful when they occurred, but they became less frequent.

The loneliness persisted. Both sons urged me to sell the house and move closer to one of them but I refused. The last thing I wanted was to become dependent, emotionally or otherwise, on my children. I would visit each of them but only for infrequent weekend stays. I was incredibly grateful for the love and support they all gave me. I remember particularly sitting on the sofa with Frances in their den. In her quiet way she got me to talk of feelings I had been reluctant to express and then held me as if I were a child when I was at last able to cry.

When the empty house became too much to bear, I began to travel. Al and I had always enjoyed traveling, independently whenever possible. It was now more practical to go on organized tours and I found that many had an educational component that made them very attractive. I took several tours to France, led by experts on the French Impressionist painters. I returned to Florence to learn more about the Renaissance.

I cruised the Volga from St. Petersburg to Moscow, seeing many of the small villages with farmhouses and huge domed churches constructed entirely of wood. The centuries, the wars and political upheavals had apparently not touched them. The tour group had arranged a private performance of the Kirov ballet in a small theater in the Winter Palace. I had seen the Kirov several times in Paris and New York but this intimate performance on their home ground was particularly memorable. We had many lectures on Russian history. I was particularly fascinated by Peter the Great. He had been tall, over 6'4", and noted for his personal modesty, his desire to modernize his country, and his love of doing things with his own hands. He reminded me of Al.

CHAPTER TWENTY-THREE

Breast Cancer

(Written for First Edition of Book, Published in 2006)

I had begun to settle into a relatively normal life when a routine mammogram revealed a suspicious density in my left breast. It was a few days before Passover and I didn't want to ruin the holidays. The whole family were planning to celebrate together in Maryland at the home of Luke and Frances. The holidays were now the responsibility of the next generation. Everyone, including Al's brother and his family, had celebrated all the religious holidays at our home when the children were small. But now we spent the autumn High Holidays, Rosh Hashanah and Yom Kippur, with Ralph and Deb, and Luke and Frances held the Passover seders at their home, in the spring. We all looked forward to these few times when we could all gather as a family and I decided to postpone the biopsy until I returned to Westfield when the holidays were over.

Debbie called to discuss holiday plans. We were having our usual logistical discussion of who would do what, where (there are so many dishes to be made for the Passover feasts that we all try to do our share). Debbie suddenly stopped in mid-sentence. "Mom, what's wrong?"

"Nothing's wrong," I lied. "What gave you that idea?"

"Mom, please tell me the truth. I can tell something's wrong." I told her.

There occurred a sudden reversal of roles. Debbie began to scold me and issue orders. "You will *not* have a biopsy in New Jersey where there is no one to care for you. And you will not postpone the procedure. I will make arrangements immediately with Dahlia Sataloff at Pennsylvania Hospital, and you will stay with us until you are well enough to go home."

Dr. Sataloff, a noted breast surgeon, is a good friend. Obediently, I followed Debbie's orders. The mass was malignant, and I had a lumpectomy. Debbie stayed with me through the entire procedure. I couldn't have received more devoted care. I had developed a genuine love for both my daughters-in-law, and hoped it was returned in kind. But Debbie's concern and thoughtfulness during this difficult time was above and beyond anything a mother could expect from her own daughter.

As soon as the incision healed, I was scheduled to start six weeks of daily radiation therapy, followed by five years' therapy with the drug Tamoxifen. Despite Ralph and Debbie's reluctance, I insisted on going home to have the radiation therapy done at Overlook. I was quite confident that the treatment there would be the equal of any university center. Lou Schwartz, the director of radiation oncology at Overlook, had come from Columbia. I had recruited him at the same time that Jim Wolff had left Columbia to become director of the Valerie Center. Lou, a brilliant and dedicated physician, had devised several methods of his own to make radiation therapy more focused and effective, thereby decreasing the trauma of the procedure.

Much has been written and there have been many media presentations on the reactions of women who are diagnosed with breast cancer. These have ranged from great courage in some to disabling panic in others, along with the "Why me?" phenomenon. Whatever the woman's reaction, the reports emphasized that the diagnosis was a major calamity in their lives.

It is difficult to explain why I felt only minimal emotional disturbance when confronted with this unpleasantness. Perhaps it was that Al's death and Ralph's illness had been so very much more cataclysmic. Perhaps it was the realization that the cancer had been caught early and there was every reason to believe it would not recur with proper treatment. Certainly the support of my family, particularly Debbie's role in facilitating the surgery and after-care, was an important factor. I had always scorned self-pity and realized what a destructive emotion it could be. I had no inclination to indulge in it now.

A short time before the end of the six-week course of radiation my grand-nephew, Diego Sanchez, the son of Barbara Ogur, Moe's daughter, planned to be married in California. I was very anxious to attend the wedding. Our families had grown apart since Moe's move to Southern Illinois. Although Moe had died following heart surgery, I wanted to see the rest of the family and renew family ties. I spoke to Lou Schwartz about missing a few days' treatment.

"Sure," he said. "It's over the Memorial Day weekend and we'll be closed anyway. Have a good time."

I still felt fatigued from surgery and radiation. My children questioned the wisdom of my traveling cross-country, but I was determined. We all decided to go. The wedding was out-of-doors in the California sunshine and everyone appeared delighted to renew old acquaintances. It reinforced my determination to take advantage of every happy occasion no matter what the obstacles.

Later that year I received a special offer from one of the touring companies to go to France on the Concorde, spend several days there, and then go by the rapid tunnel train to London. It was close to Debbie's birthday and I asked her if she would like to go with me, as a birthday present. She was delighted.

I had not enjoyed Paris since Al's death but seeing it now with Debbie brought back only happy memories. We had lunch on a Bateau Mouche, the sightseeing boats on the Seine. I showed her where Al and I had had our memorable picnic. I took her on our own private, regrettably limited tour of the Louvre, showing her my favorite paintings. We stayed at the Hotel Internationale, between the Place Vendome and the Rue Rivoli, just around the corner from the famous French couturier houses. We did a little shopping and a lot of looking. In London, we toured the city and went to a different show every night. Debbie has a beautiful voice and relaxes from her strenuous schedule as an obstetrician by singing in community musicals. She loves the theater and seeing those London shows with her was a special treat. I had never enjoyed giving a birthday gift more.

CHAPTER TWENTY-FOUR

Fifty Years in Medicine: What a Change!

(Revised for Second Edition of Book, Published 2009)

B en Spock had once told me that in order to win honors and respect, all you had to do is survive long enough without getting senile. He was certainly right. I find now that when I speak occasionally at a meeting or conference, no one argues with me. It is most disconcerting.

A whole series of honors and awards come with age but sometimes the most meaningful ones are not accompanied by plaques, silver trays, or certificates. My grandniece, Rebecca Sinclair, the daughter of Moe's son Jonathan and his wife Marie, asked me to "hood" her when she graduated medical school in Virginia. The hooding ceremony at medical school graduations goes back to medieval times and acknowledges the new status of graduates as members of the profession by placing a hooded velvet mantle on their shoulders when they receive their diplomas. The ceremony is usually performed by the dean or president of the college unless the recipient has a family member who holds the same degree. I was greatly honored that Rebecca asked me to do this and suddenly realized that she represented the third generation of women in our family who had become physicians. Moe's daughter, my niece Barbara Ogur, is now a professor of medicine at Harvard.

I thought a great deal about how medicine had changed between Rebecca's generation and mine. Women in medicine are now much more accepted: the harassment and bias I had to endure without complaint are now illegal. But some forms of discrimination still exist. There is a disproportionate number of men in the higher ranks of

FIFTY YEARS AS A PHYSICIAN

I "HOOD" MY GRANDNIECE, REBECCA O. SINCLAIR ON HER GRADUATION FROM UNIVERSITY OF VIRGINIA MEDICAL SCHOOL

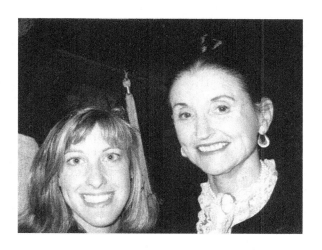

I HAVE A SERIOUS CONVERSATION WITH MY FIRST GREAT-GRANDNEPHEW, REBECCA'S SON, DAVID SINCLAIR

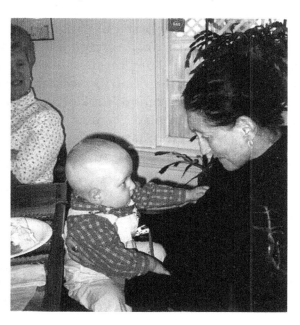

237

academia. It is difficult for women to rise above a certain level in faculty appointments and there is still bias in the reimbursement of women who do the same work and have the same responsibilities as men. However, the number of women in medicine, which was less than 4 % in my generation, is now approaching 50%.

My years of training were difficult, but I think that young doctors have an even more difficult time today. We did not have all the technology and medications that are available now. When a sick person stopped breathing, we said they expired. That term literally means "to breathe out" (the opposite of inspire, "to breathe in") but we used it as a term synonymous with death.

Today, even lay people are trained in CPR (cardiopulmonary resuscitation). Patients who stop breathing not only have basic CPR, but are often intubated, shocked to restore heart function, and subjected to innumerable invasive procedures to resuscitate them. Young doctors work unceasingly under great stress to keep patients alive. I do not deride these advances in intensive care. They have saved many lives. Sometimes, however, the philosophy of "that patient is not going to die on my watch" gets carried too far. It's as if death is a disaster that must be prevented at all costs, and was not the eventual outcome for all mortals.

On the fiftieth anniversary of my graduation from medical school in 1998, the college honored our class during graduation ceremonies by having us sit on the stage and be introduced individually to the audience. The president of the college listed our accomplishments and the contributions we had made to medicine. The graduation ceremony took place in the Academy of Music in Philadelphia, a place I knew so well. Before the ceremonies our class was given a special room near the stage, the Eugene Ormandy room, where we could rest, renew old acquaintances, and don cap and gown. Looking at my classmates, I realized that many seemed old and infirm. It was depressing. I was having difficulty recognizing some. But as we greeted one another, memories came flooding back, and I remembered faces as they used to be.

One was Patricia Borns, now a professor of radiology in Philadelphia. Pat and Eva Reich had come to vacation with me at Schroon Lake following our graduation from medical school.

The three of us had gone skinny-dipping off a deserted island in the middle of the lake. I had taken some pictures of Pat and Eva. One day, many years later, Ralph was going through some old albums and came across the pictures. He opened his eyes wide. He recognized Pat immediately, even sans clothes. "Why, that's my professor of radiology!" I made him promise never to tell her he had seen the pictures.

Eva Reich was not there. I hadn't seen her in many years. She had visited us several times after I married and had met Al and the children, but I had never been able to return her visit. I sent her a note urging her to come to the reunion. She had not answered me, but she had sent her regrets to the school, saying that she felt too old and frail.

Not seeing Eva was a great disappointment. She had spent a very turbulent life. She had remarried and had a daughter whom I had never met. She had started a family practice in Maine near her father's research center at Organone and had spent part of her time helping him with his research. Then Wilhelm Reich was sent to federal prison. I never really understood why. I believe it had something to do with his obtaining radioactive materials, used in his studies of the orgone theory, without the permission of the federal government. Reich died in prison and Eva was greatly affected. She became the trustee of his estate, "the keeper of the flame." Nagged by feelings of persecution about the way he had been treated, she continued her rebellion against organized medicine and practiced in a way that got her into difficulty with the Maine Medical Society. She quit practice. The last I heard from her, she had been traveling worldwide to talk about her father's theories.

All the other members of the class who attended had lived busy, productive lives. Some were still active in private practice or academia. Most had retired. We admired pictures of children and grandchildren. As soon as the obligatory photos of our class had been taken and greetings exchanged, I went to visit my family, who had reserved seats in the front of the auditorium. We stood talking together until we heard the signal that the processional was about to start. I raced back to join my class but was stopped by an usher.

"I'm sorry, ma'am" he said, "but this area is reserved for the fifty-year graduates."

"But I am a fifty-year graduate" I protested. He frowned in disbelief and I began to laugh. "Young man," I said, "you have just made my day."

Our class walked down the aisle in solemn procession. When we reached the stage, young undergraduates were stationed to assist each of us up the few steps to the platform. As I accepted the outstretched arm, I suddenly felt the irony of the situation. I had just returned from climbing the steep Inca ruins at Machu Picchu, high in the Andes, and now it was assumed that I needed assistance to climb those few steps.

When it was my turn to be introduced, I saw my family smiling and applauding. It was one of the proudest and happiest days of my life.

The progress that has been made in medicine since I graduated medical school has been nothing short of spectacular. The common childhood diseases, such as measles, mumps, chickenpox and whooping cough have been virtually eliminated by immunization. So have *Hemophilus influenza* infections which could cause not only a deadly form of meningitis, but also an infection of the windpipe called epiglottitis, a form of croup. Viral croup occurred more commonly and was not as dangerous as the bacterial form, but it was sometimes difficult to distinguish from epiglottitis without taking an X-ray. The thin, moveable leaf-like epiglottis which forms the lid to the windpipe becomes enormously swollen and looks like a big fat thumb. Its movement is compromised and there is the danger that it will completely obstruct the windpipe making it impossible for the patient to breathe.

When I first started practice, the only way to treat epiglottitis was by tracheotomy, cutting a hole in the obstructed windpipe below the epiglottis and inserting a tube so that the patient could breathe again. I think that I dreaded this disease more than any other that occurred during the winter months. Because it could be difficult to differentiate between viral croup and epiglottitis if X-ray facilities were not immediately available, failure to make the proper diagnosis could be drastic. When a child is having great difficulty breathing there often isn't enough time to reach a hospital before death occurs. All pediatricians of my generation were instructed in the technique of doing an emergency tracheotomy, but we never performed it on a living creature during pediatrics training.

There is a common myth that a tracheotomy is easy to do. Many Hollywood movies used to portray a heroic family doc saving a child's life by doing an emergency tracheotomy on the kitchen table with a penknife. Nothing could be farther from reality. During my residency, I had seen a skilled surgeon who had been inadequately trained in doing this procedure on a child accidentally cut one of the large blood vessels surrounding the trachea. He could not control the bleeding in time to save the child's life.

Later, it was found that children with epiglottitis could be treated by intubation (inserting a tube through the nose or mouth past the swollen epiglottis into the windpipe) to establish an airway. Once they could breathe, the emergency was over. We had the time to give antibiotics and steroids to diminish the inflammation. But it was still a fearful disease until immunization against the cause, the bacteria *Hemophilus influenzae*, became available.

One night when Ralph was about three years old, he woke with severe croup. He was having trouble breathing and was very frightened (as were his parents). I dreaded the idea of taking him to the hospital. The doctors in the emergency room had less training than I in performing a tracheotomy on a child. Al constructed a steam tent around his bed and crept into it to be with him.

"Make believe we're camping out" he said to Ralph, with a huge grin. To me he said quietly, "You've got your emergency equipment, right?" I nodded, unable to speak. I had a kit to do an emergency tracheotomy but I hoped never to use it, least of all on my own child.

"I doubt that we'll need it, but let's have it up here just in case," said Al.

I got the kit and put it by the bedside.

"Try to get some sleep," said Al. "I'll call you if we need you."

I dozed fitfully, going into Ralph's bedroom frequently to check how things were. Towards morning, both Ralph and his father were sleeping peacefully in the tent and I breathed a special prayer of thanks.

Epidemics with poliomyelitis occurred every summer and parents were in constant fear that their children would be affected. Once, a mother brought in her child who could not move her right leg. The mother was in panic because she felt the child was paralyzed with polio. The child did not appear that ill, although she was crying inconsolably. I gently examined the leg and felt a foreign body embedded in the muscle. I could grab the two ends between my fingers and move it back and forth. I told the mother, "Annie doesn't have polio, she sat on a needle and it's in her thigh." The mother looked at me unbelievingly. We took an X-ray of her leg. It showed the sharp outline of the needle including the eye. We removed it with instant cure.

There are many more immunizations available today. The viruses for Hepatitis A and B had not yet been discovered when I was in medical school. They can now be prevented with vaccines. These viruses can cause liver failure and cancer, which are no longer threats to the immunized child. Other forms of hepatitis still exist, but progress has been made in eliminating them as well. There is now a pneumococcal vaccine that prevents the meningitis, the recurrent ear infections, and the pneumonia we used to see frequently. There is also a vaccine against meningococcal infections. Meningococcal meningitis was formerly the most common cause of meningitis, and we saw it frequently. It is much less common today.

Vaccination against smallpox used to be routine but we stopped using it when the last case of smallpox was recorded, and we thought that it was eliminated from the entire world. It is unfortunate that with concerns about bioterrorism, we have to consider using it again.

Many parents are disturbed by the number of immunizations recommended for their children, and articles have been published about their side effects, the risk of autism, etc. Most of these media blitzes are sensationalist, without scientific proof.

The warnings given by TV and Internet "experts" have been thoroughly discredited. While it is true that all immunizations carry a certain degree of risk, it is minuscule compared with the risk of contracting the disease they were designed to prevent. When England responded to a media blitz and stopped giving whooping-cough vaccine, the number of deaths and complications rose astronomically over the next several years and they resumed immunizations.

Parents used to consider the contagious diseases of childhood as rites of passage, and were amused rather than alarmed when their child came down with measles, mumps or chickenpox. Complications were rare and the general public did not know these existed. But when you consider how common the childhood contagious diseases were (every child eventually got most of them) you will understand that many hospitals saw critically-ill children suffering from the complications every year. I have seen children die of measles—and chicken pox—encephalitis, and I have seen many more brain-damaged. The fact that we can now immunize our children against these diseases is a great blessing.

Polio immunization has also saved many children from death or profound disability. The Children's Specialized Hospital, with which the Overlook pediatrics service was affiliated, used to be called the Children's Country Home. It was filled with children paralyzed by poliomyelitis, some unable to breathe without the aid of an "iron lung," a primitive type of respirator for older children and adults. When I first started practice, I made daily rounds there. By that time the number of polio cases had decreased and the hospital was admitting patients suffering from many different types of neuromuscular diseases, such as cerebral palsy. One Fourth of July in the 1960's we were planning to go on a family picnic but I felt that I had to make my rounds before we left.

Our children groaned in protest but I assured them I'd be back within the hour. The hospital was just a short distance from our house, less than 10 minutes away. I was racing through routine rounds when an emergency code was called. One of the children was having a convulsion. I ran to his bedside and found that seizure activity was still continuing and he was profoundly cyanotic: a deep shade of blue. Ordering oxygen and anticonvulsant medication, I put my finger in his mouth to clear the airway and could feel a strange substance in his throat. I hooked my finger around it and pulled it out. It was a big piece of hot dog obstructing his airway. He took a deep breath, the cyanosis disappeared, and he stopped convulsing. I had a long talk with the dietary department. They swore it was not part of his diet. One of the other children who was ambulatory and had attended the Fourth of July barbecue at the hospital must have given him this special treat to share in the celebration. I was only a little late for our own holiday activities.

Operations on the heart were unheard of when I went into medicine. There was an almost religious taboo concerning heart surgery. When an operation on a child's heart was successfully performed at our hospital in the late 1950's we were wild with excitement and felt that a new era in medicine had begun. The operation was not actually on the heart but on a patent ductus arteriosus, a duct between the main artery leading from the heart, the aorta, and the pulmonary artery. This communication is normally present in every fetus, but should close spontaneously after birth. When it does not, it is sometimes necessary to operate. Today, surgery on a patent ductus is considered a relatively minor procedure and the success rate is close to 100%.

Operations on a wide variety of congenital heart diseases including the blue-baby syndromes are now done routinely. Children who would never have been able to live a normal life are now laughing and playing with their friends as if nothing had ever been wrong. Columbia has a large series of successful heart transplants in children. The diseased heart is totally replaced with a new one. These procedures often involve profound ethical dilemmas. There are many more patients in need of heart transplants than there are children's hearts available. Painful decisions have to be made. The whole field of medical ethics has expanded greatly and is now an integral part of the curriculum in medicine.

Medical advances have also effected many changes in the treatment of cancer. People are always wishing for a cure but different cancers have different causes. I compare it to wishing for a cure for fever because it is that unspecific. You have to know the reasons for the disease and attack the causes. The field of molecular biology is doing that. This basic research has a long way to go but has made impressive progress. This has resulted in great strides in the treatment of many childhood cancers. When I started practice, the diagnosis of leukemia was a death sentence. Today, over 70% of all childhood leukemias are cured. The percentage is even higher for the most common type, acute lymphoblastic leukemia

I had several children in my practice develop leukemia. I made one of the diagnoses looking through the microscope in our downstairs laboratory, the same microscope my parents had bought for me when I started medical school. I remember staring down at the leukemia cells on the blood smear under the microscope, dreading the idea that I had to go upstairs and tell the mother what I had found. It would still be difficult to tell a parent such news today, but I could offer much more hope.

Other forms of cancer that have undergone impressive improvements in treatment are brain, kidney, and bone cancers. One day, the mother of one of my patients came over to me while I was shopping at the supermarket and told me she was worried because her little boy had started to limp. "He hurt his leg sliding into home base during a Little League game the other day," she said, "but the limp seems to be getting worse."

I said, "Bring him in this afternoon. I'll have a look." When I examined him, I could feel a tender swelling in his leg. "It's probably an injury from that ball game," I said, "but let's take an X-ray to be sure."

As soon as I saw the film developing in our X-ray room downstairs, I knew that something was terribly wrong. When I put the film into the final wash, I kept bobbing it up and down in the crazy hope that I could wash away what I was seeing. I went upstairs and said to the mother, "There's something on the X-ray that should be seen by an orthopedist. Which one do you use? I'll call him and try to arrange for him to check it out right now."

On the phone, I told the orthopedist what I suspected, and sent mother and child over with the X-ray film, still wet, in its frame. He called back less than an hour later.

"You're right," he said, "it looks like an osteogenic sarcoma."

"Yes," I said, "I just didn't have the heart to tell her. I would much rather have you do it."

"Thanks a lot," he said, sarcastically.

At that time there were few survivals from that form of cancer. Today, with newer forms of treatment, we can hope for a cure. The little boy lived less than a year.

Probably the most dramatic advances in pediatrics have been made in the care of the high-risk newborn. These are babies born prematurely or with infections, breathing problems, jaundice, and anemia due to blood incompatibilities between mother and child, or other difficulties. I frequently had to do exchange transfusions on babies born with an Rh blood type that was incompatible with the mother's blood type. Now, a simple shot given to the mother has eliminated the problem.

Infant mortality when I started practice was between twenty and twenty-five per thousand. Now it is about six per thousand. There is an entirely new field of pediatrics, neonatology, that has its own sophisticated technology and knowledge devoted to the care of the high risk newborn. When I was director and first asked for a neonatologist who would come just for a few hours each month to train our pediatricians and residents in some of the most basic new methods of intubation and resuscitation, the administrator laughed and said he had never heard the term, neonatology. He considered it a new-fangled fad not worth the hospital's investment, and the request was denied.

The nursing staff came to my aid. Mary Lindner, at that time head of nursing for obstetrics and the nurseries (she later became director of nursing for the entire hospital) learned that a course was being given at the University of Medicine and Dentistry in Newark, to train nurses in neonatal intensive care. It was directed by Dr. Shyun Sun, a neonatologist who had trained at Columbia. Mary went to take the course herself and then sent each of her nurses in turn to be certified in intensive care. It soon became apparent that our nurses knew more than our doctors, a situation that could be very embarrassing for the hospital. With some reluctance and hesitation, I was granted money for new nursery equipment. The hospital also agreed to pay for Dr. Sun's workshop at Overlook, held once a month, to train the pediatrics staff.

Mary and I were delighted. Mary had the engineering department paint us a sign reading Neonatal Intensive Care Unit. We hung it over the door to one of the rooms in the nursery where we had concentrated all the new equipment. And so the NICU, the Neonatal Intensive Care Unit, at Overlook was officially created.

We have learned much more about the toxic effects of environmental substances. Lead used to be used in most paints and lead poisoning was common in small children who would chew on peeling paint chips, or whose parents repainted a second-hand crib with a lead-based paint. Most of these sources have now been eliminated. By law, lead in paint is now restricted to only a very few specialized products. We have eliminated lead from gasoline, so that we do not breathe in exhaust fumes laden with lead. But there is still lead in the environment. In the New York Times of March 27, 2004, there was an article about unsafe lead levels in the drinking water of the District of Columbia. The pipes that carry the water are very old lead pipes. City officials blame the federal government for ignoring the danger and the city has fired the head of the Health Department because they believe he has not adequately responded to the problem. We have found that the concentration of lead in the blood that we once thought acceptable (that is, the amount in the blood was too low to have a deleterious effect) is now considered unacceptable. Even though obvious signs of toxicity may not exist, these small levels have been found to affect the ability of children to coordinate and integrate knowledge. These are subtle disabilities that can only be diagnosed by sophisticated tests. Even small concentrations of lead can affect a child's ability to learn. As far as I am concerned, the only acceptable level of lead in the blood is zero.

I once had a patient who came in with symptoms that made me suspect lead poisoning. His blood lead level was not very high and, almost as an afterthought, I asked the laboratory to test for other heavy metal toxicity. The levels of mercury in his blood were astronomical. I tested all the other members of his family, but none had elevated blood levels of mercury. No one knew when and where he could have been exposed to mercury. I kept questioning the family for clues, like a detective on the hunt. I finally learned that this two-year-old had been "helping" his father paint the bottom of their boat at the seashore. I had the paint tested. It was a special anti-fouling paint used to prevent the bottom of boats from becoming encrusted with barnacles. It was loaded with mercury. With the proper treatment, the child recovered.

Advances in all these fields have had a dramatic effect on the care of children and has improved the prognosis for many serious diseases but progress has been even greater in adult medicine. I experienced a dramatic example of this just a short time ago. I was attending the college graduation from Brown University of my grand-niece, Mara Sanchez, when her stepfather developed severe chest pain at the Friday night dance preceding the weekend graduation. He was rushed to the hospital, where cardiac catheterization revealed that one of the coronary arteries of his heart was obstructed. Damage to the heart muscle had not yet occurred. They inserted a stent, an object that could be threaded through a catheter into a blood vessel leading to the heart. It opened up the obstructed coronary artery. He was released from the hospital in time to attend Mara's graduation that same weekend.

The doctors had cautioned him to remain seated in a wheelchair during the graduation but we found him standing on line at the buffet after the ceremony. With much urging he reluctantly agreed to return to the wheelchair. Turning to me he said, grinning, "Gloria, what would you have said if, at the beginning of your career, they had told you that the events of this weekend would be occurring during your lifetime?"

"Michael," I said, "I would have considered it crazy science fiction." I thought ruefully of my father who had suffered with chest pain for years, had become a cardiac cripple and had died because there was no treatment for these heart problems.

One of the most recent advances that would have been called "science fiction" has been the increasing use of the portable defibrillator, a very simple device that could save the lives of 50% of people who have heart attacks outside the hospital. It is recommended for use in airports, gambling casinos, gyms and other public places. I'm sure that its popularity will continue to grow. Any lay person can use it after a minimal amount of training. I recently read of a project to train sixth grade students to use it. They were just as efficient as adults.

This chapter doesn't begin to summarize the progress that has been made since I started to practice medicine. It is just an attempt to recount some of my experiences with the changes that have occurred. Not all changes have been good. Many infectious diseases can now be treated effectively, but new ones have taken their place. AIDS continues to kill millions of people. It can be prevented, and there are drugs available to treat it, but that requires the appropriation of staggering amounts of money. At the World AIDS conference recently held in Barcelona, it was estimated that $10 billion would be required annually to control the AIDS epidemic. The amount of money available, particularly in undeveloped countries, is pitifully inadequate

Because antibiotics are often used inappropriately, many infections are now drug-resistant. When I started training, there were no drugs for tuberculosis, and many people died. Then a whole series of drugs to treat TB were discovered, and the prognosis improved considerably. Now many strains of the tubercle bacillus have become resistant to treatment and the death rate from this disease is climbing again.

New drugs, before they can be released for clinical use, have to go through stages of testing for their safety and their efficacy. Their possible interaction with other drugs has to be considered. This prolonged period of testing is very costly, and pharmaceutical companies must show a profit. They often find that it is not cost effective to obtain the data that these drugs are suitable for use in children. This deprives children of the benefits of many new drugs. We call them "therapeutic orphans."'

Despite all the progress we have made, we are now beset with new problems. The health care system in the United States is the most expensive in the world. Our health care costs per person are greater than any other country. But we are the only wealthy, industrialized country that does not provide all citizens with health insurance. Medical expenses are the principal cause (60%) of personal bankruptcy in our country. Although we spend more money on health care, our infant mortality rate is greater than 31 countries ranked by the World Health Organization (WHO). Our infant death rate is 6.26 per 1,000 live births: most other countries, including Ireland, Portugal and Slovenia have rates between 3 and 5 per 1,000.

The WHO has also developed a measure called healthy life expectancy (HALE) that indicates the number of years a newborn can expect to live a healthy and productive life. Japan leads with an average of 75 years. Twenty-seven other countries are better than us, including Australia, Greece, United Kingdom, Italy, Germany and France. WHO in 2000 ranked the US health care system 37th in overall performance, right next to Slovenia, and 72nd in overall health among the 191 member nations included in the study.

Surely our country, which considers itself the leader of the free world, can do better than this. The debate over health care reform is presently one of the principal issues facing Congress. Many are concerned over the costs of the various proposals, but the costs, to our economy and to our health, of doing nothing are even greater. I could list, as can every other doctor, the obstacles in obtaining approval for the funding of our patients' care from insurance companies and HMO's. For those who worry about the government coming between doctor and patient, the obstacles that presently exist are of even greater concern, because of the profit motive and the huge salaries and bonuses paid by these private organizations.

The health and well-being of every citizen should be of the highest priority in any democracy. Since I was a child, I have heard every proposal for social reform opposed as a form of "socialism". I recall the heated arguments in my own family when FDR introduced Social Security. My father, a rugged individualist, was dead set against it, influenced by talk that it was a government hand-out: a form of socialism. But it was this Social Security that helped my Dad in his old age and made my widowed mother economically independent. No one today would dare call for the elimination of this program because it was "socialism." The same holds true for Medicare, signed into law by LBJ in 1965. This also faced opposition on the grounds that it was "rampant socialism" fostered by the federal government. Yet some of the most heated opposition to health care reform today is from folks who don't want the government, which created and administers this program, "messing around with their Medicare."

It comes down to the matter of trust. I believe that the present administration, having the same ideals as the administration that created Medicare, can be trusted to protect the interests of our senior citizens. This country is now led by a president who had many opportunities to establish a lucrative career in private law practice, but decided instead to become a community organizer when he graduated law school. His example has inspired many young people to become more active in the affairs of this nation. I believe that the majority of our citizens have recognized President Obama's manifest concern for their welfare and have given him an electoral mandate that will help solve some of today's problems, not only in health care, but in many global issues as well.

CHAPTER TWENTY-FIVE

The Grandchildren

(Written for First Edition of Book, Published in 2006)

L ike all proud grandparents, I think my grandchildren are very special. They are a remarkable bunch of kids, each a unique individual with different strengths that become more apparent as they grow older.

All of the children have attended or are attending Jewish day schools. It was Al's wish that they know more about their religion than we had learned, and his sons have respected that wish. I had never been enthusiastic about a parochial education, but when I saw how the children flourished in small classes with dedicated teachers, I changed my mind. Neither Debbie nor Frances come from religious homes, but they too have been delighted with both the secular and religious aspects of their children's education. Most important to me has been their pride in their heritage. As a child, I could not relate to the children at Schroon Lake or in the city. Those feelings of alienation continued into adulthood. It is good to see my grandchildren happy and secure with their identity.

Joshua and Benjamin, the two oldest, are Ralph and Debbie's sons. Josh was born on February 16, 1988 and Ben on December 23, 1991. Both remember Al, though Ben was not yet four years old when he died. Josh had a very close relationship with his grandfather, and was very sensitive to my difficulties at the time of his death.

Josh, now a teenager, is quiet and uncommunicative unless he's discussing sports, when he erupts with excitement and enthusiasm. He is a natural athlete with a roomful of trophies in soccer, basketball, ice hockey, baseball, and Lord knows what

THE GRANDCHILDREN

BIRTH OF MY FIRST GRANDCHILD, JOSHUA D. SCHRAGER
FEBRUARY 16, 1988

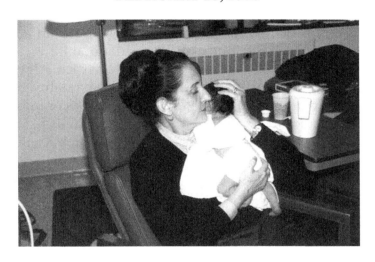

JOSH AND HIS BROTHER, BEN, 2004

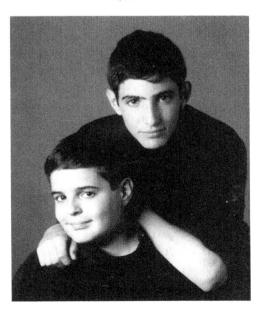

else. He also has a beautiful voice and is presently a member of the Keystone State Boychoir. He has toured Cuba twice, as well as Russia, Germany, South Africa, and the western United States.

When Josh graduated elementary school, a Jewish middle school had not as yet been formed in his area, and so he transferred to Abington Friends', where he is presently attending high school. Initially I was concerned how he would adjust to this new environment, but with his athletic abilities and his beautiful voice, he made new friends quickly, particularly because he has such a thoughtful and sympathetic personality.

Ben is as communicative as Josh is not. He has opinions and impressions about everything, which he never fails to express, sometimes leaving us speechless. He has a quick intelligence and a marvelous sense of humor, does very well in school, and is an avid reader. He is a particularly affectionate, loving child, and despite the usual rough-housing and sibling rivalries, it is quite apparent that he and his brother are very devoted to each other. Like Josh, he has a beautiful voice and is also a member of the Keystone State Boychoir.

One of Ben's first concerts with the choir was at the inauguration of the Kimmel Center in Philadelphia during the holiday season of 2001-2002. The boys were scheduled to sing in the atrium, which extends upwards for several stories and is surrounded by balconies on each floor. It was an imposing sight for young boys, especially since, in addition to the seated audience, all the balconies were lined with spectators looking down to hear them sing. The boys stood in several rows on their temporarily-constructed grandstand. The sun shone down from the top of the atrium and hit the group like a strong spotlight. It became very warm. Suddenly, one of the boys in the top row fainted, toppling forward onto the boy below, creating a domino effect. Some spectators immediately rushed forward to assist, and I followed behind them.

It always amazes me that the first instinct of untrained people is to make a fainting person sit up and drink water. This is not very physiologic. It is important that they lie flat, or at least sit with their head between their knees if there is no room to lie down, so that the head is lower than the heart and adequate oxygen can reach the brain. We carried the boy away to an inconspicuous corner, and a member of the choir staff came running up. I said, "I've been through this before. In a group that has been standing for a long time, if one faints, others are sure to follow. You'd better get out there and catch them as they fall." Before long, we were ministering to six fainting boys. They recovered quickly and a few were able to return to the choir for their solos. Ben had not fainted. Although most of the songs were Christmas carols, his solo was from *The Prince of Egypt*. When he sang the chorus of the song in Hebrew, many members of the audience began to clap rhythmically with the music. I was very proud of him, and also of the choir directors, Joseph Fitzmartin and Steven Fisher. The choir is a mixed ethnic and racial group, and it was good to see several different religions and traditions represented.

Elana and Alexander are Luke and Frances's two children. Elana was born February 1, 1995 and Alec on September 27, 1997. Elana, my only granddaughter, is my soulmate. She is very beautiful, with long chestnut hair reaching below her waist. Her interests certainly correspond to mine. We are both passionate about ballet, and Elana at the slightest opportunity will dance, twirl and do arabesques with or without musical accompaniment. She reads incessantly, and has been known to finish an entire book in a day. She is as athletic as her cousins, is an excellent swimmer, and joins the boys in climbing trees and balancing on walls when we picnic. She loves beautiful clothes. When I travel, I always try to bring back something for the children. It is always easy to find something for Elana: a doll dressed in native costume, or a hand-embroidered dress. Try as I might, it is much more difficult to find interesting things for the boys. They often end up with T-shirts.

Alec was born after Al died and is named for him. His features are very different from my other grandchildren. They all have dark, wavy hair and dark eyes. Alec has very straight, sandy hair with reddish glints, just like Al's. I also think that his eyes, light gray-green, are like Al's, but in truth they are probably more like his mother's. He is a thoroughly delightful child with an infectious grin that is ready to appear at the slightest provocation. I have

LUKE, FRANCES, ELANA, ALEC AND I
VISIT WASHINGTON
2003

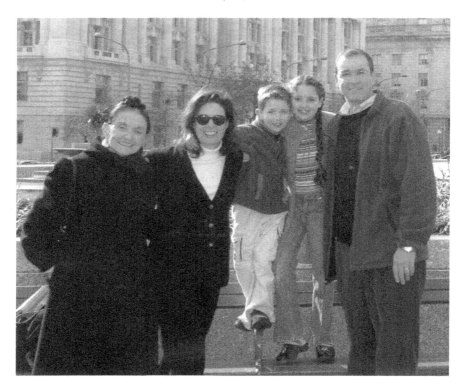

pictures of all my children on my refrigerator door. When I look at them each morning, it helps start the day right. I must confess that the one that makes me smile the most is a picture of Alec when he was much younger, with that marvelous grin, spaghetti hanging out of his mouth and sauce spread all over his face.

Alec always seems to be playing some variety of ball. I saw him recently in a soccer game. It was on a day when I drove down to Bethesda for the weekend, and arrived about noon after a four-hour trip. Luke and Frances urged me to rest and skip seeing Alec's team play that afternoon, since I "might not enjoy the sight of little kids fumbling a soccer ball." Of course I went, and it certainly was worth the effort. Alec scored all eight of his team's goals. I shouted myself hoarse cheering, but after the fourth goal thought it might be more tactful, out of respect for the other parents, if I just signaled my delight with a "thumbs-up" sign. Alec looked at us after each goal, grinned, and gave me a "thumbs-up" in return.

The four grandchildren are very close, and love to visit one another. In addition to the religious holidays, we try to schedule some vacation time together, though this is often difficult because of conflicting work and school schedules. Josh, who now spends his summers as a junior counselor in a camp, is always willing to play with his younger cousins, and they adore him.

CHAPTER TWENTY-SIX

My Life Today

(Written for First Edition of Book, Published in 2006)

I t would be wrong to say that one gets used to loneliness. More accurately, one adjusts to it and begins to prefer it to the alternatives. After Al's death, I met several men through friends, family or on trips. None of these friendships lasted very long. Well-meaning people lectured me on the futility of comparing other men to Al. Their lectures were similar to Eva Reich's psychoanalytic diagnoses of my problems with commitment to a serious relationship while I was in medical school. I listened politely but saw no point in continuing friendships I did not enjoy.

On my 75th birthday I went camping in Yosemite with Luke, Frances and Frances's extended family, including all their offspring. It was my first visit there and I was greatly impressed by the spectacular scenery and the waterfalls. One day they all decided to climb Sentinel Dome which looms over the valley. Luke was dubious about my ability to make the climb, but I assured him I would go as far as possible and if I tired I would simply wait by the trail until they returned. I climbed without too much difficulty to the rocks that formed the summit. I have developed some balance problems and decided that climbing over the rocks to the top with nothing to hold on to was not a good idea. I was reluctant to ask for help since everyone was burdened with children of various ages in backpacks, astride shoulders, etc. I sat down on a rock to wait.

Frances's brother, John Marshall (former chief counsel for the Lake Tahoe commission), called down from the top, "Hey, Gloria, you're not going to quit on us now!"

I shouted back that it was balance, not exhaustion, that made me stop. He came leaping down the mountain as sure-footed as a mountain goat, and helped me to the summit. It was an exhilarating moment with the falls and the valley spread out below us. Laughing and shouting, we took a bunch of group pictures, and then everyone sang "Happy Birthday." I couldn't think of a more wonderful way to celebrate my 75th.

In the summer of 2001 we joined Frances's French cousin, Fabienne, and her family in Europe. Fabienne is one of the most beautiful women I know. She has two teenage daughters, Emmanuelle and Severine, who resemble their mother. The year before, Fabienne had thought it would be a good idea for them to spend a year in American schools, to become more proficient in English. Severine stayed with Luke and Frances, and Emmanuelle with Frances's brother John and his wife Kate. We became very fond of both girls and when they returned home, we decided that we would all spend the following summer in a rented villa in the south of France. They could not find one large enough to accommodate all of us, but Claude, Fabienne's friend, came to the rescue. Among his wide circle of acquaintances was an Italian woman of royal ancestry, still called "The Princess." She has a villa in a small town in Tuscany near Siena and she invited us to stay there.

The villa was at the top of the mountainous little town of Sinalunga, near the cathedral. The exquisite Tuscan countryside spread out before us like a scene from a Renaissance painting. The villa had at least three floors, possibly more, filled with antiques and art that had been in the family for generations. In the back was a private garden with a pool and a gaily striped tent for lounging in the shade.

We took frequent day trips to explore the countryside, visiting Florence, Siena, Pisa, Lucca, and many small towns whose names I've forgotten. It was the time of the Palio, the traditional horserace that dates back to medieval times. It is conducted with much pomp and ceremony, the participants in medieval costume. Although the Palio in Siena is the most famous, similar contests occur in other towns as well. We were having dinner in Montepulciano, a neighboring town, on an evening when they were inaugurating their Palio with a torchlight parade. We could hear the drums echoing off the ramparts which surround the town, and joined the procession of people who trailed at the end. As the parade broke up we found that some of the magnificently costumed and bejeweled young men were quite enthusiastic about having their pictures taken with Emmanuelle and Severine. Those two were much admired wherever we went and more than one night's sleep at the villa was disturbed by young men serenading them from the street below. I told Luke and Frances that I felt I was living in a foreign movie.

We met Princess Alessandra. I think my granddaughter, Elana, was a bit disappointed. She expected her to arrive with gown and tiara, possibly drawn in a golden coach. Instead, she came in shorts and crash helmet on her motorcycle. She was a vivacious young woman and we spent a day with her in Florence, where she conducted us on a private tour and arranged for a leisurely lunch at one of the outdoor cafes. Elana and Alec were absolutely marvelous, and adapted with good humor to the erratic schedule of their elders. I had been concerned that they might be too young for this type of travel, with jet lag and the inevitable fatigue and dislocation, but they held up like troupers. Italy was a wonderful country to travel with children: they were constantly getting special treats from waiters and storekeepers, which certainly increased their good nature.

It was some time in 2001 that I started writing memoirs. I had never really given the idea much thought, but Frances in her gentle way insisted that this history was important for future generations. She said that my grandchildren, particularly Elana, should have some concept of the difficulty women had in achieving equality. The project started modestly enough, but with Frances's suggestions the book soon took on a life of its own. I consider her my muse.

I don't travel as frequently as I used too. I still swim a mile each morning and play tennis at least once a week, and now work out in the JCC gym with a trainer. My former independent workouts became a little too enthusiastic, which resulted in some tendon injuries. A personal trainer who can monitor one's efforts is a good investment for the long run.

These activities almost ended permanently in the autumn of 2003. Every morning I run down the stone steps of our front porch to get our daily copy of *The New York Times*. I didn't realize that the first frost of the autumn had occurred the night before and the steps were coated with a sheet of ice. When I put my foot on the first step, I slipped and plunged heavily to the cement walk below. A fall down six stone steps can be disastrous to a woman over seventy years old. I felt gingerly for broken bones and to my relief found that both arms and legs were working fine. But the bottom of my left pant leg was torn and saturated with blood. We live in a quiet residential neighborhood and there was no one on the street that early in the morning. I couldn't just lie there, bleeding profusely. In desperation I crawled back up the icy, slippery stairs, grimly holding on to the railing. I limped to the kitchen, made a pressure bandage out of an old towel to stop the bleeding, and called Charlie and Ros Neustein who rushed over in their car. Charlie is a pediatrician and together we examined the injury. I had a deep, uneven gash in the front of my left leg. It had formed a flap, folded back to expose the bone underneath. The edges of torn skin were ragged and dirty.

Charlie said, "We've got to get you to an emergency room."

I said, "No way. This leg needs a plastic surgeon."

I called Dr. Jerome Spivack, who is a good friend. He said, "I'll meet you at my office immediately."

It took him almost an hour to get my leg back together again. When he had finished and the leg was nicely wrapped, I looked at him tentatively and said, "Jerry, the Neusteins and I have tickets to the Met this evening to see "La Juive." I'd hate to miss it. Do you think it would be okay if I went?"

My surgeon, who has removed several skin cancers from my face, knows me well enough not to be surprised at my little eccentricities. He just answered calmly, "I don't think it would be a good idea. You should keep your leg elevated and I want to see you again tomorrow."

I said, "I'll keep it elevated for the rest of the day, and also when riding into New York on the back seat of the Neustein's car. I may even be able to keep it elevated in the opera house. How long do you think the local anesthetic will last?"

He answered resignedly, "Until about the middle of the second act."

He was right. Going to the opera that night was not the thing a sane person would do. I developed some complications that probably could have been avoided if I had acted sensibly, and my leg took a long time to heal. Yet I feel it was worth it. "La Juive" is a wonderful opera and the production was excellent. I'm sorry that it is rarely staged today. It was Enrico Caruso's favorite opera and the last one he performed before his death.

Debbie looked critically at my healing wound and boasted, "Your scar is not as impressive as my scar."

I retorted, "That's because I had a plastic surgeon sew it up and you didn't."

Debbie's accident occurred the year before when she and Ralph were on a cruise in the Caribbean. Their boat had anchored off a small island and Ralph had gone fishing. Deb had stayed behind to water ski. She fell and the ski rope tore a deep gash in her thigh, from knee to groin. The boat had a nurse on board but no doctor. The nurse paled when she saw the wound and said, "I can't handle that. We'll have to airlift you to the nearest hospital."

Debbie, in her cute little bikini, said cheerfully, "That's not necessary. I'll sew it up myself. I'm a doctor. What kind of equipment do you have?"

The nurse answered apologetically, "Little more than a first aid kit. But I do have a local anesthetic, some black silk skin sutures and a needle."

Debbie reassured her, "I'll manage fine." Sitting on deck while a bunch of passengers watched in fascinated horror, she injected a local anesthetic and then calmly sewed up the torn muscles and skin with the black silk. Her only concern was that she was using non-absorbable sutures that would remain deep in the muscle and could not be removed. "Oh well," she thought philosophically, "I'll worry about that when we get home."

The plastic surgeon at her hospital looked at her leg admiringly. "A damn good surgeon sewed this up."

"What about the black silk in the muscles?" asked Debbie.

"Don't worry about that," he said. "We often had to use non-absorbable sutures in the army. They'll just sit there. They won't cause any trouble."

When Al was alive, I was supremely uninterested in our finances. He urged me to become more knowledgeable but I was always impatient with such details. I didn't even balance my own checkbook. "Just make sure," I told him, "that there's enough in my account so that my checks don't bounce."

Now I have to manage not only my everyday expenses but make decisions about investments and estate planning. I've been very fortunate in getting excellent advice from David Schiller, Debbie's brother, a lawyer who helped me through the legal tangles of settling the estate. Alan Achtel, a good friend, helps me with estate planning and remembers the details much better than I do. Both Luke and Ralph, neither of whom ever bothered with money matters, have also become much more responsible. Luke in particular has become astute about investment strategies. I have benefited from his advice, but have occasionally lost an opportunity through negligence in acting promptly.

One day, returning from my early morning swim and workout, I remembered Luke's recent telephone call and decided to phone Joyce Fischman, who handles my accounts at Smith Barney. She said quietly, "The stock market is closed."

"But Joyce," I protested, "today isn't a holiday."

She said, "Two planes have just smashed into the World Trade Center. You'd better put on your radio or TV."

That was how I found out about the events of September 11, 2001. Westfield is a small town but it has a significant number of people who commute to New York City to work. Eight of them died in the World Trade Center disaster. I knew the families of some. Several neighbors had close escapes due to late trains and missed connections. The tragedy was deeply felt by the whole nation but the towns surrounding the city felt a personal loss with an immediacy that affected us all.

Many doctors called to volunteer their services. Luke, who had worked a year in the Emergency Department at Bellevue Hospital, called from Maryland and spoke to their director. "I'm leaving right now to drive to Manhattan. I can be there by early afternoon."

"Sorry, Lew, that won't be necessary. Most of the people were killed. We have few wounded to treat."

When I went into the city to teach at Columbia the next day, Pennsylvania Station in Manhattan was crowded with soldiers in fatigues patrolling the area. Trains were running on schedule but the atmosphere was tense. I reached the hospital on time but one of the doctors I work with was very late. Her subway train had been stopped and had stood between stations without explanation for a long time before proceeding. The rumor had spread that Penn station had been attacked. I wondered how I was going to get home and we checked the latest news on one of the computers. The rumor was false but the subways were delayed because of precautions. If unclaimed packages were seen, the trains were stopped until they could be removed.

A short time later both Ralph and Luke came to visit with their families and we went to Liberty State Park on the New Jersey side of the Hudson River, to look across at lower Manhattan where the twin towers had stood. Smoke was still rising from the tragic gap in the skyline. I took some pictures and put them into an album next to pictures I had taken from the same spot, the windows of the twin towers golden, reflecting the sun setting in the west over New Jersey.

But life goes on despite grief, anxiety, and frustration. I take particular pleasure in my grandchildren. When Josh and Ben went to South Africa to perform with the Keystone State Boychoir, a small group of parents organized a parallel tour. Initially Ralph could not arrange his schedule to go but they asked Debbie and me to go as staff physicians. We were delighted.

Almost as an afterthought, I checked to see if my malpractice insurance would cover me and found that it would not. The insurance company would not even consider a rider to the policy. Debbie found the same true for her insurance carrier and we were strongly advised against taking on medical responsibilities without malpractice coverage. We were disappointed, but decided to go as simple tourists. Things worked out for the best. Ralph was able to organize his schedule so that he could join us, and we were able to enjoy the trip without having any medical obligations.

South Africa is a very beautiful country. We went in July, their winter season. We dressed in layers against the morning chill but we were peeling off jackets and sweaters by noon. The weather was very mild; it was an ideal time to visit. We were taking malarial prophylaxis, and had packed all kinds of insect repellants, but I didn't see one mosquito in all the time I was there.

The safari we took in Mala Mala, a private game preserve, was particularly exciting. Hunting in not allowed, and the animals totally ignore humans since they do not regard them as either a threat or as prey. We were safe as long as we sat quietly in our Land Rovers, and we were able to get within a few yards of lions, leopards, elephants—the whole galaxy of animals one would see in a zoo. But here it was completely different, because we were on their turf. We saw lions stalking water buffalo. The herd suddenly became aware of the enemy and all turned to face in that direction. Powerful male buffalo ringed the outside with the more vulnerable members of the herd in the middle. It was a standoff since lions think twice before attacking full-grown male buffalo, who have dangerous horns.

We witnessed the drama of a leopard, crouched on a rock above a water hole, waiting for some impalas to come within striking distance. He knew he couldn't outrun them and the impalas, knowing he was there, never came close enough for him to pounce. They kept circling because of their desperate need for water. This, also, was stalemate.

We came within a few feet of a lioness lying in the sun on a rocky plateau nursing several cubs. I was amazed that our presence did not disturb her at all, and it was a delight to see the cubs tumbling over each other in play when they had finished their meal. The mother would swish her tail back and forth and the cubs would stalk it and attack it ferociously. She seemed to be having as much fun as her babies.

One day we inadvertently found ourselves in the center of a herd of elephants that had suddenly appeared, crossing the trail around us. This was not a good spot to be in and Greg, the ranger who was driving, stepped on the gas to get out of there in a hurry. One of the female elephants considered us a threat and attacked. I knew we were in trouble when our Zulu tracker, who sat in the back of the open vehicle and was usually very taciturn, began to yell wildly in Zulu. Between his shouts, the trumpeting of the elephant and our headlong flight through the brush, the next few moments were unforgettable. We held on for dear life. It wasn't until later, when the elephant had given up the chase, that I realized how hard my heart was pounding and had collected my wits enough to recognize that we had been in real danger.

We learned a lot about the politics of South Africa and the struggle against apartheid. We were supposed to visit Robben Island, where Nelson Mandela had been imprisoned for many years. But the surf was too rough that day and all small boat outings were canceled. We spoke with many different people about South Africa's history, the present, and the future. We found everyone friendly and articulate. One of our guides was an Afrikaaner who gave her version, but that evening when she wasn't present we went on an unscheduled tour. Our native bus driver gave us an entirely different perspective. His people were proud of their struggle for independence, with which we could certainly sympathize and identify. But his attitude about treatment for AIDS, shared he said by most of his countrymen, distressed me greatly. Although two of his sisters had died of the disease, he felt strongly that South Africa should not become dependent on other countries who offered to supply the necessary antiviral drugs at little cost. His argument was that the infected people were going to die anyway. Prolonging their lives with expensive drugs and medical care would be an unacceptable drain on the country's struggling economy. I tried to argue that treatment could halt the spread of the disease, particularly from pregnant women to their newborn babies, but he was adamant. He was ready to support education and the use of condoms for prevention, but nothing else.

The highlight of the trip was the concert, in which both Josh and Ben had solos. Four different choirs performed, the first three South African. One was all-white male, the second all-white female, the third all-black of both sexes. Our Keystone State choir was last. When they appeared, the children representing every creed and color, and began to sing God Bless America in their pure childish voices, I was overcome with emotion and pride in our country.

I had planned to take a trip to France that year but canceled it. As much as I love that country, I find their present foreign policies reprehensible. The wave of anti-Semitism that has spread through France, the burning of synagogues and the desecration of cemeteries brings back memories of Kristallnacht and the era before WW II. The fear of terrorism will not deter me from taking other trips or in altering my life in any way. I will not allow that strategy to succeed

I teach at Babies Hospital, now called The Morgan-Stanley Children's Hospital of New York, once a week. Dr. John Driscoll, former director of neonatology, is now Chairman of the department. I have always considered him a good friend. The atmosphere at Columbia, reflecting the personality of the Chairman, a great, good-natured bear of a man, is warm and friendly. Dr. John Truman, a former director of pediatrics at Morristown Memorial Hospital, which is a neighboring institution to Overlook in New Jersey, is now Physician-in-Chief at Columbia, working with Dr. Driscoll. Our friendship goes back many years to the time when we were faced with similar problems in developing residencies in community hospitals. We find that we still have many interests in common, particularly a fascination with the history of medicine.

A group of retired faculty, organized by Dr. Solomon Cohen, has formed a special teaching service that keeps us busy. My contacts with medical students and the resident staff stimulate "the little gray cells" that Hercule Poirot, Agatha Christie's famous detective, talks about, to function more actively. These bright, delightful young people seem to laugh a lot even when discussions get heated and challenging. Since I have more free time than the full-time faculty, I have the luxury of reviewing cases in depth, emphasizing the importance of a detailed history and physical examination. The students seem to appreciate this leisurely approach and ask endless questions. I often feel I learn more from them than they from me.

Another great attraction at Columbia is the book club formed by Dr. Rita Charon, that has expanded into a program in Narrative Medicine. This involves both students and faculty in the humanities, and increases the sensitivity of the physicians to the problems of their patients. We read both American and foreign literature, including poetry, and our perspective and understanding are enhanced by discussions with both the authors and people of different backgrounds. Rita has greatly influenced my writing and my thoughts about my medical practice.

LIFE TODAY

TEACHING AT COLUMBIA

Retirees Use "the Luxury of Time" To Teach

An unusual group of individuals have joined the ranks of CPMC volunteers: they are retired pediatricians who spend a half day or more a week in the Pediatric Emergency Room teaching medical students, interns, and residents.

The group evolved from an experience Solomon J. Cohen, MD, had early in 1997. After attending a conference at CPMC, he sat in the ER listening to students, residents, and attending pediatricians discuss cases. When the ER started to get busy, the Attending asked him to lead the discussion. "The Attending needed to be productive and efficient," Dr. Cohen says. "I had the luxury of time with students. I could sit and talk for an hour about one case."

Ever since, Dr. Cohen has spent a day a week in the ER, and he has recruited other retirees so that at least one is on hand Monday through Friday.

"It's a marvelous way to keep up your skills and interests," says Gloria O. Schrager, MD, a former Director of Pediatrics at Overlook Hospital in Summit, New Jersey, who teaches at P&S. "Most residents, interns,

and medical students are superbly trained in the latest knowledge and techniques, but they haven't related yet to patients. We teach them how to help children and their parents handle anxiety and how to examine a child in a nonthreatening way, adapting techniques to the age of the child. We try to teach the art of medicine and the clinical judgment that comes from long years of experience."

Dr. Cohen, who practiced

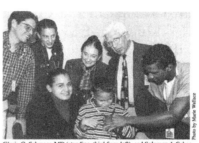

Gloria O. Schrager, MD (standing, third from left), and Solomon J. Cohen, MD (second from right), teach in the Pediatric ER. A patient, Garibaldy Carmpagna, demonstrated his proficiency with a stethoscope to his mother (seated), and (standing, from left) interns Bill Olcott, MD, and Elyse Olshen, MD, and (far right) Sean Yetman, a third-year student at P&S.

in Westfield, New Jersey, for 42 years and also teaches at P&S, says, "We like, at this point in our lives, to feel useful. And these interns and residents are very sharp. It's great fun to be with them."

For Elyse Olshen, MD, an intern in Pediatrics, "It's nice to have doctors with so many years of experience. They emphasize the fundamentals—taking a history, doing a thorough physical exam." Another intern, Bill Olcott, MD, says, "I admire the doctors

who are so dedicated to the field that they spend their free time teaching us."

Other participating pediatricians are Josephine Kerr, MD, Ruth Donovan, MD, Bert Grossman, MD, Alvah Weiss, MD, and Donald Eisenstein, MD. Drs. Kerr, Donovan, Grossman, Eisenstein, and Cohen completed residencies at CPMC.

According to Dr. Cohen, the group members bring a total of approximately 280 years of experience to their teaching.

THE FAMILY CELEBRATES MY 80TH BIRTHDAY
JULY 11, 2004

THREE GENERATIONS OF WOMEN PHYSICIANS:
MY NIECE, BARBARA OGUR, MD
AND MY GRANDNIECE, REBECCA O. SINCLAIR, MD

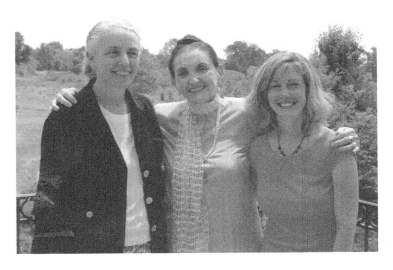

MY SONS, RALPH M. SCHRAGER, MD AND
LEWIS K. SCHRAGER, MD AT MY 80TH BIRTHDAY PARTY

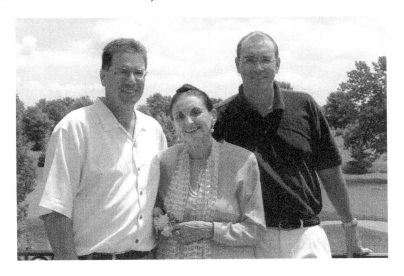

THE KEYSTONE STATE BOYCHOIR SERENADES ME ON MY 80TH BIRTHDAY

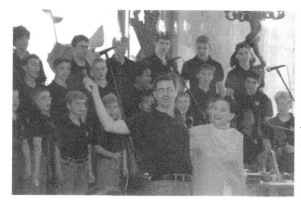

Steve Fisher, Associate Director, leads the choir

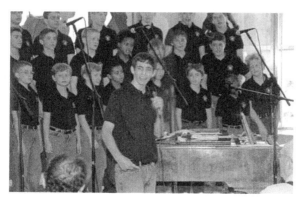

Josh does his solo

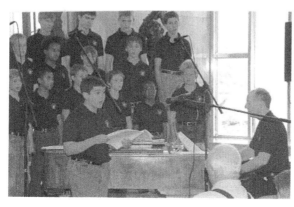

Ben does his solo Joseph Fitzmartin, Director, at the piano

I now have time for all the hobbies I once admired but couldn't fit into my life. I garden a great deal, and do a lot of baking. Before each Sabbath I bake chalah (the special Sabbath bread), and apple pies, and share them with my dear friends, Charlie and Ros Neustein, when we have a Sabbath meal together. Sometimes I take them to my children if I visit on a weekend.

My children insisted on having a party to celebrate my 80th birthday on Sunday, July 11, 2004. Initially, I was somewhat reluctant about the idea. I don't hide my age, but I don't broadcast it either. But our friends and family are now scattered over many different states, literally from California to New England, and we rarely have a chance to see one another. Any excuse to have us meet for a happy occasion would be welcome. I was delighted that just about everyone came, though many had to travel long distances.

Although it was not a surprise party, I was astonished by the amount of effort and thought my children had expended. Ralph and Deb had organized it in an old manor house in Philadelphia, and over fifty people were present. Luke had borrowed many of my old picture albums and he and Frances made three large poster displays: the first entitled "Family Life—Part I," devoted to pictures of my childhood in Schroon Lake; the second, "A Doctor's Life," depicting my professional career; and the third, "Family Life—Part II," portraying my marriage to Al and the different phases of our family's growth since that time. Everyone seemed fascinated by the pictures, and they must have really been paying attention, because later, after the dessert course of the Sunday brunch, my sons hung up a huge "Jeopardy" game, with various categories devoted to my life, interests, and family. Most of the questions were very funny and the group, divided into four teams, competed with much excitement and laughter. (One example: "The candidate for President of the United States who survived eating Gloria's oatmeal." Answer: "Who was Dr. Benjamin Spock?") There must have been over a dozen children present, and the little ones scurried around distributing the points to the winning teams. All the kids—grandchildren, grandnieces, grandnephews—then joined me in blowing out the candles on my birthday cake. The youngest toddler, David, my great grandnephew, began to sob because he couldn't get close enough to blow, so we lit them again to give David his turn. His beaming face was one of the highlights of the day.

I thought that nothing could equal the excitement and delight of that morning, but more was to follow. Later in the day, the Keystone Boychoir surprised me, at an impromptu concert, by singing "Happy Birthday", and both Josh and Ben sang solos. Then, the following Tuesday, Ben sang the boy's solo with the Philadelphia Orchestra when they performed the new "Lord of the Rings" symphony at the Mann Music Center. The solo was at the end of one of the movements, and the entire audience rose to applaud and cheer. It was truly a memorable time.

And so my days are full. I drive down to visit my children in Philadelphia and Bethesda frequently, but keep these visits short. All of us have busy lives, and short visits are best.

I had resigned myself to a tranquil old age, but the state of the world today will not permit that. I have fought for certain goals all my life and find that I must continue the fight now for the most important goal of all—a peaceful, secure world for my grandchildren.

THE NEXT GENERATION

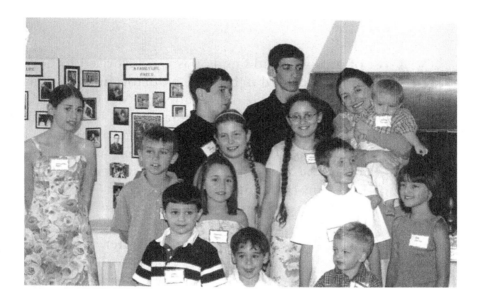

CHAPTER TWENTY-SEVEN

Comments of Barbara Ogur, MD

Assistant Professor of Medicine
Harvard Medical School
Niece of Dr. Schrager

M ost of my extended family was not surprised to hear that I had decided to become a doctor. In fact, it was not portrayed to me as much of a challenge. My aunt Gloria had already proven elegantly that a woman could both have a medical career and raise a family. Perhaps that is one reason I looked for my own challenges as a woman and as a woman physician. And I found them in the turbulent upheavals of the era in which I lived my early adult life.

My parents certainly did their best to hard-wire me to become a doctor or a scientist. I remember early on being taken to a movie about Marie Curie, the Nobel prize winner, and being encouraged to believe that intelligent women could do much for the world by pursuing careers in the sciences. My father, whom I worshipped, told me bedtime stories about the wonders of modern science. And the whole family contributed to the mythology that I was the next Gloria, my father's younger sister who had become a doctor. Older relatives often called me "Gloria" by mistake, a slip I could never understand. I never thought there was any resemblance between my tall, poised, self-assured aunt and my slightly chubby, fuzzy-headed self.

I was raised in Carbondale, Illinois, a small town in southern Illinois, home of Southern Illinois University. My father, Gloria's older brother Maurice (Moe) Ogur, moved there from Brooklyn, New York, in an attempt to save his career in Microbiology and his family from the ravages of McCarthyism, after having refused to testify against politically-active friends from the Brooklyn College of the activist 30's and 40's. Carbondale was (and still is) a sleepy, southern town of about 20,000, over 100 miles from the nearest city, St. Louis. The schools had no tradition of academic achievement. There were no bagels, no Seltzer water, few Jews. The schools, movie theater, and restaurants were segregated until the mid 60's. My schoolmates had never seen a curly-headed, swarthy-toned little girl like me. Jews, as I was told many times, were the killers of Christ. And in an environment where girls and young women were valued for blonde good looks or perky, cheerleader personalities, my intellectual achievements and quiet reflectiveness set me aside as a nerdy outcast. I found refuge in books and in the beauty of the surrounding foothills of the Ozark Mountains.

Fortunately, a family friend suggested that I might be very happy going away to Radcliffe College. I, of course, had never heard of it. My preference was to attend the University of Michigan or the University of Wisconsin.

My high school, however, had very little experience in helping students go away to college. Most students ventured no farther than S.I.U. or the University of Illinois. As a result, my Michigan and Wisconsin applications did not get processed correctly, and, despite my all A's and 99th percentile SAT scores, I was not admitted to either one. My only acceptance was to Radcliffe College.

I arrived at Radcliffe a total backwater hick in 1965, one year before the beginning of the maelstrom that was the 1960's on college campuses. Despite my lack of urban worldliness, I felt I had found a home. There were intellectuals, finally, and Jews from New York City, seeming to me like long-lost cousins. We embarked upon an intense exploration of every facet of the adult world we were poised to join. In 1966, anti—Vietnam war protest began in earnest at Harvard, and I joined a sit-in against Dow Chemical Company. When I went home and told my parents about it, my father stayed up with me late into the night, telling me the story of his early political activity, a secret from everyone in Carbondale. While I never could fully appreciate the fear which drove him to flee New York in the 50's, I knew my father to be a strong, brilliant and outspoken person. Although his revelation about his past was intended to make me cautious in my activism, it had a mixed effect. I found myself more and more drawn towards the idealism of transforming the society to a more just one, as if my inner soul was singing the music of my parents' youth: the Weavers, Pete Seeger, and union songs.

Although I graduated from Radcliffe College as a pre-med major, my mind was much more on the revolutionary change I believed was occurring in society and on building a home and family in a more egalitarian, communal model. I rejected the idea of taking up any of the roles I saw in traditional society, and went off to California to look for a new world. I baked my own bread, lived in a commune, hung out with a struggling rock band, tried to learn Yoga, and fell in love. But when the turbulence of the 60's and the turbulence of my post-adolescent personal life came together to make me feel lost and confused, I returned close to the very path my parents had envisioned for me. I decided, at the breakup of a relationship, that since I would never be able to have the family life I was seeking, I could at least be of service. So I applied to, and was accepted at my state medical school, The University of Illinois in Chicago.

I was not, however, finished with political activism. In medical school I joined the Student Health Organization, a group of students involved in anti-war activities and also in promoting access to health care for all. Our activities ranged from protesting racist or sexist speakers and policies of the school, to promoting education on disparities in health, to doing screening projects in inner city neighborhoods in conjunction with various community groups, to working in free clinics in poor neighborhoods. I worked on a project to do health screening in one of the large housing projects on Chicago's south side, where I went door-to-door with a member of the Black Panther Party.

I remember going from one apartment to another: one meticulously clean with a matching living room set carefully covered with plastic, the next with children dressed only in diapers on a dirty mattress on the floor. I carried away a deep sadness for the damage our divided and unequal society has caused, and a commitment to continue to work to help those who suffer its effects. To that end, I applied for a residency in Internal Medicine at the hub of health care activism in Chicago, Cook County Hospital. County was the safety-net hospital for the city, the last resort for the sickest and poorest. While other hospitals still got away with "performing a wallet biopsy" before offering treatment, County refused no one. With the sheer volume of admissions, and the lack of access of most of our patients to outpatient preventative and early diagnostic care, our patients came in severely ill and with a wide range of illness. I look back on those years at County as a time of intense learning and intense camaraderie, as those of us who chose to work there came with a strong sense of mission.

Nor was I finished with my pursuit of family. During these years, I fell in love with another medical student, a handsome, politically active Puerto Rican. We impetuously rushed into having children, while caught up in finishing medical school, residency, and political activism. In fact, I arrived at my internship in July, in Chicago, at County, an ancient relic of a public hospital with 20-bed wards and no air conditioning, in my 6th month of pregnancy.

I remember dragging my big belly up to the bedside on rounds in the 90 degree heat and having the patient exclaim, "Doc, sit down, please!" It never occurred to me that having (and then raising) a baby and going through the physical and intellectual demands of the residency might be overwhelming. From this vantage point, I look back in awe, and also with some regret. I certainly became the master of efficiency. My husband and I managed the routines of child-care, the handing off of Diego to his grandmother at all the crazy hours that residency required. We even found moments of quality time. I remember always finding a way, even coming home late after 36 hours of non-stop work, to have an hour of playing or reading a bedtime story. And I marveled at the achievement of every baby milestone, even if I wasn't always present for them.

I was a member of one of the first classes in medical school to admit large numbers of women: our class was about twenty percent female. So I was not alone in trying to combine career and family. I recall an editorial in one of the medical journals at this time, in which a prominent clinician proposed that women needed to stop whining about the difficulties of combining career and family, and to go out and hire some help so we could get on with it. This occasioned my first medical publication: an angry letter to the editor asserting that there was a real difference in the experience of a child raised by nannies and one who has the concentrated love and attention of its family.

The next phase of my life was to be a phase of career and family. I had taken two years to complete my third year of residency in order to spend time with my son, Diego.

I had my daughter, Mara at the completion of my last year of residency, and went to work in academic ambulatory primary care clinics, first in Shreveport, Louisiana, then at the University of South Florida, in Tampa, Florida. But, ironically, just when I was finally trying to put together a more planned and orderly life for the sake of my children, my life was once again swept up in the turmoil of the times. My husband "came out" as bisexual in 1982, just as the first reports of immune deficiency illness in homosexuals were coming out. We divorced and remained friends until his death from AIDS in 1992.

At this point it became clear to me that I would not have Gloria's life: the loving two-career, American family that the middle-class women's movement idealized. I would have to create a new kind of family, and try to limit my pursuit of career to give me time to function as a single mother. At the same time, medicine has always been a refuge from the problems of life for me. No matter what is going on in one's personal world, patients command full concentration and commitment on the job, and thus bring one out of oneself. So I discovered that I derived strength and perspective from continuing in the work I loved.

I moved to Cambridge, Massachusetts with my children for my dream job: a primary care physician in a community health center affiliated with the Cambridge Hospital. Cambridge Hospital is a Harvard Medical School affiliate with a strong mission to provide health care to the under-served. Having studied Spanish intensively during my residency, I have taken great pleasure in developing sufficient skills in the language to enable me to communicate with patients from Central America, the

Caribbean, and, more recently, new immigrants from Colombia. In 1988 and 1989, I participated in two delegations to the war zone of El Salvador to bring medicines and food, and to bear witness to the conditions in the homeland from which so many of my patients were fleeing. It was my first exposure to victims of war, and my first view of life in the third world. The first night of my first trip, a weeping mother came to us with her baby in her arms. He had infant diarrhea, which had already killed her first 2 children in a refugee camp in Guatemala. Now he was too weak to suck and dying of dehydration. We were a 6-hour hike from the nearest hospital. A nurse midwife and I sat and spooned rehydration fluid into the baby's mouth, and he survived. The brief experiences of that visit gave me insight into the worlds of my patients, which, I believe, allow me to better understand them.

In 1988 I attended a 3-week training in HIV care in San Francisco. I carried home the unforgettable vision of room after room of emaciated, dying young men at the AIDS hospice, and returned to participate in the formation of a multi-disciplinary AIDS team at the Cambridge Hospital. For the next 12 years I practiced part-time in general internal medicine, and part-time in HIV primary care. As for many HIV care providers in those early years, my work in HIV care was also a means of coping with the tragic decline and death of my children's father. I tried, as much as possible, to help my children find ways to become constructively involved in helping in the battle against HIV disease, hoping that they, too, might find a way to give creative or productive outlet to their feelings of pain and loss.

In recent years, in addition to practicing primary care, I have become more involved in the development of innovative curricula. Medicine has been an enormously involving and rewarding career for me. Those rewards have come from the inseparable combination of the intellectual challenge of understanding and applying medical science and the essential interpersonal connection with the patient, without which the best diagnostic and therapeutic thinking is often useless. The goal of our curricular work has been to ensure that students learn both of these critical aspects of the profession. Our work has culminated in a pilot Longitudinal Integrated Clerkship which is being implemented in Cambridge this year.

I remained a single mother for 13 years. I was blessed with bright, healthy children, who, despite the losses and tragedies of their lives, are positive, funny, loving people, who have truly been the joy of my life. We have shared many wonderful times together: bedtime stories, Friday night pizza and videos, trips in the car singing oldies or listening to books on tape, weeks in August on the Cape, winter vacations to the White Mountains or the Caribbean. Nine years ago I remarried, and have found in my husband, Michael, a loving companion who both challenges me to keep thinking and growing and also supports me in my efforts and my dreams. With him by my side, my life feels dramatically easier and sweeter.

My students frequently ask my advice, particularly about when and how to combine career and family. I find it difficult to answer. Certainly my personal life did not turn out as I had planned, and my career has been interrupted by losses and family responsibilities. In the end I have had a life which combines both, although not as elegantly or smoothly as Gloria's. Life brought many surprises, and I know that life will continue to bring its surprises. Perhaps my experiences will help me provide support for young women whose pursuits of career and family do not, whether by choice or by surprise, follow a traditional path. I hope to find the strength to continue to learn from the hard times and to treasure the joys of both career and family.

CHAPTER TWENTY-EIGHT

Comments of
Rebecca O. Sinclair, MD

Dr. Schrager's Grand-niece

W hen my great-aunt Gloria asked me to write about my life as a woman physician, I was honored and touched to make my contribution to her memoir. I do not remember the exact age when I decided to become a doctor, but I know that I made the decision when I was very young. The many physicians on both sides of my family served as positive role models, and this certainly was a great influence. In particular, Great-Aunt Gloria and my Aunt Barbara were wonderful examples of strong, brilliant women who balanced rewarding careers with rich family lives.

In addition to the physicians in my family, my parents were pivotal in my decision to pursue a career in medicine. They instilled in me the confidence to accomplish any personal or professional goals that I would set for myself. As a result, I became an empowered young woman who believed that one person could make a difference in the world. They also taught me the importance of making a contribution to our community, and helping the many less fortunate individuals in our society. This idealism and altruism helped shape my career aspirations.

My nuclear and extended family members did not demonstrate gender differentiation in their hobbies, intellectual pursuits, or career paths. I took this upbringing for granted until I later met women who were not given the same support by their families. These women were instead left feeling that they could not balance family and career. I did not consider these restrictions when making my personal and professional choices, although I did encounter gender bias later on in my training. particularly when it came time to have children.

After completing my undergraduate studies at the University of Virginia, I entered the Medical College of Virginia. My class was a unique blend of people from varied backgrounds, including a priest, an astrophysicist, and a professional tennis player. Women comprised approximately thirty percent of my class, which was less than the national average of about fifty percent at that time. We had an unusually large number of married students, and a total of thirty children were born during the four years of our studies. I felt a great deal of pride in this heterogeneous group who each brought a unique life experience to the class. These people were committed to their studies and to their patients, and were able to simultaneously maintain fulfilling personal lives. My experience at MCV was an extremely positive one. I felt I received an excellent education in the sciences, as well as a superb introduction to clinical medicine.

I met and started dating a wonderful person in my class during my first year of medical school. He was kind, sensitive, easy-going, and intelligent. Jeff Sinclair, who became my husband and soul-mate, has been a huge part of my success as a woman physician. He has always valued my professional life as much as his own, and we have each made sacrifices for the other at different stages of our demanding training and careers. We were married during our fourth year of medical school, and Jeff and I began the complicated process of "couples' matching" in residency programs: trying to choose and be chosen by training programs in the same geographical location. We were matched by our first choices, in Philadelphia: I in Internal Medicine and Jeff in General Surgery.

I started my Internal Medicine Residency at Temple University Hospital as an energetic and compassionate young physician. The hospital was in a tough area in North Philadelphia and provided care to a very sick patient population. Resources were limited and the residents and staff were overworked. It was an excellent place to receive strong clinical training by caring for patients with a challenging range of pathology and psychosocial issues. I put in very long hours at the hospital, and struggled to maintain my idealism by focusing on the patients for whom I was caring, but it was hard not to get discouraged. I found I had to develop a harder "shell" as a survival technique. During this time, I became pregnant and encountered some of the gender bias that still exists in medicine. But nothing could dim the delight accompanying the birth of our first son, David.

When I finished my residency, I accepted a position as a Geriatric Fellow at Abington Hospital, where my husband was doing his fifth and final year of surgical training. While I had no intention of practicing geriatrics exclusively upon the completion of the fellowship, I felt the additional year would be beneficial in light of our aging patient population. The hours were reasonable and we were able to spend more time together. I became pregnant with our second child and we began to make plans to relocate to Virginia, where our friends and families lived. We both loved growing up there and missed the close family relationships.

We jumped at a wonderful job opportunity for Jeff in a Virginia suburb south of Washington, D.C. He joined a surgical practice whose colleagues shared his priorities: they valued their careers but also valued time with their families. I decided to delay my job search since I was due with my second pregnancy. Shortly after moving, we experienced the joy of having our second son, Matthew.

Jeff and I do not have the traditional division of labor that many couples have adopted. We have developed a "teamwork" approach to addressing everything from the most mundane household tasks, to raising and caring for our children. I know that many women with careers are still expected to do all the work at home, including the primary responsibility for their children. Some of these women feel frustrated and overwhelmed, and consider leaving their jobs. I respect that this is an extremely personal decision that each woman must make, but it is helpful to share the process with one's spouse, and have his support.

A close friend from medical school offered me a position in his private practice, but I remained committed to a career in indigent care. After doing some networking, I got some leads from people who had powerful connections in community health and I have helped organize and am now the Medical Director of a Primary Health Care Van Project. Working out of a mobile van, we provide medical care to an uninsured, indigent population. I have a true passion for the work I am doing, and find the challenges of working with this population extremely rewarding. We are funded by the State of Virginia and a series of grants. The number of people we serve has grown each year. I was recently honored by receiving the 2005 Humanitarian Award at the annual dinner of the United Way of the National Capital Area.

Women physicians have come a long way in many respects since the time my great-aunt Gloria bravely faced challenges on every level. My generation takes for granted the fact that women can pursue a career in medicine and now comprise almost half of medical school classes, though gender barriers still exist in the area of maternity leave and child care. Each woman has to figure out a balance that works for her. Support from family, spouse and partners at work are the key ingredients for success. Great-Aunt Gloria and Aunt Barbara are excellent examples of this. But it is pioneers like my great-aunt who have made it possible for the rest of us. Each of the women doctors in our family has chosen an area of medicine devoted to teaching and helping underprivileged people. I feel proud and honored that I am carrying on that tradition.